Hygiene Evaluation Procedures

Approaches and Methods for Assessing Water- and Sanitation-Related Hygiene Practices

Astier M. Almedom,[1] *Ursula Blumenthal,*[1] *and Lenore Manderson*[2]

[1] London School of Hygiene and Tropical Medicine, Keppel Street, London WC1E 7HT, United Kingdom

[2] Australian Centre for International and Tropical Health and Nutrition, University of Queensland Medical School, Herston Road, Herston, Brisbane, Qld 4006, Australia

INFDC
LONDON SCHOOL OF HYGIENE & TROPICAL MEDICINE
unicef

ISBN No. 0-9635522-8-7

Library of Congress Cataloging-in-Publication (CIP) Data Applied for.

Table of Contents

List of Boxes

List of Tables

List of Figures

List of Diagrams

List of Plates

Acknowledgements

Thanks are due to all the study teams who contributed to the development and field testing of this handbook. In Kenya, we would like to thank Tom Mboya, Veronica Moraa, Christian Odhiambo, and Zilpah Ouma (SHEWAS Project); in Tanzania, Mahalia Adamu, Adelina Chang'a, Peter Chuwa, Hashim Ibrahim, Vedasto Jalves, Mustapha Mbughu, Asha Msengwa, Stephen Mwendi, and Samuel Shaaban (WAMMA); in Ethiopia, Seble Beyene and Tsegaye Haile (GIBB/SEURECA and WSSA); in India, Anila Kumary, Kochu Rani Mathew, Lalachan, Lissy Paul, B. Manoharan, C. K. Nagesh, K. N. Nisha, K. Suresh Babu, Harish Kumar (KWA, Socio-economic Units), and Vijayalakshmi Ammal (Independent Consultant), and in Afghanistan, Abdul Qayeum Karim, Hayatullah Niaz, Abdul Hai Sahar and Shireen Sultan (BBC-AED Project) and Anne-Marie Wangel.

We would also like to thank those who provided financial and moral support to the above teams: Nancy George (ARUNET), David Adriance, Bud Crandall, Iskandar, Richard Odero, B.E.N. Okumu, Josiah Omotto and Beat Rohr (CARE Kenya), and Shoa Asfaha (CARE UK); Catherine Johnson, Julie Jarman, Saad Makwali, Brian Mathew, *Mzee* Pullinga, Ian Westbury, and Saada Westbury (WaterAid UK and Tanzania); Neil Chadder (GIBB/SEURECA, Ethiopia); Jens Bjerre (DANIDA, India) and Balachandra Kurup (Kerala Water Authority, Socioeconomic Units, India), Gordon Adam and John Butt (BBC-AED Project, UK and Pakistan); Victoria Ware and Marion Kelly (ODA, HPD).

We have benefitted from those who commented on an earlier draft of this handbook: Pete Kolsky, Sandy Cairncross, Simon Cousens, and Sharon Huttly (LSH&TM); John Pinfold (WaterAid, Uganda); Elena Hurtado (Consultant, Guatemala); Nancy Balfour and John Muturi (Environmental Health Programme, AMREF, Kenya). In particular, the peer-reviewers: Sarah Murray Bradley (Consultant, UK), John Gaskin (Sir Alexander Gibb & Partners Ltd., UK), Gillian Hundt (LSH&TM), Eva Kaltenthaler (Hallam University, UK), Harish Kumar and the Kerala study team mentioned above (Kerala Water Authority, Socioeconomic Units, India), Rose Lidonde (UNDP-World Bank, RWSG-EA, Kenya), Jane Moore (Consultant, UK), Yusaf Samiullah (ODA, Engineering), Darren Saywell (GARNET, UK), Shirazuddin Siddiqui, Shireen Sultan, Abdul Qayeum Karim, and Hayatullah Niaz (BBC-AED Project, Pakistan) and Simon Trace (WaterAid, UK) provided us with constructive and exciting ideas most of which were incorporated into the final manuscript. We are grateful to them for these and other suggestions which will be taken up in the dissemination of this handbook.

Many friends and colleagues have provided us with practical support and assistance in the production of this handbook. We would especially like to mention Caroline Smart, Rosetta Brown, and Nick Truefitt (LSH&TM), Alexander de Waal (African Rights, London) and Jenny Cooper (ACITHN, Brisbane, Australia).

This publication was financed by the Overseas Development Administration of the UK Government (ODA), Health and Population Division. The International Nutrition Foundation for Developing Countries (INFDC) and UNICEF also contributed towards the publication. UNICEF is supporting the handbook's distribution and dissemination including its translation into French and Spanish.

List of Abbreviations

ACITHN	Australian Centre for International and Tropical Health and Nutrition
AED	Afghan Education Drama, a BBC Project
AMREF	African Medical Research Foundation
ARUNET	African Research Utilization Network
BBC	British Broadcasting Corporation
CARE	A non-governmental international organization
DANIDA	Danish International Development Aid—Government of Denmark
EHP	Environmental Health Programme (London School of Hygiene and Tropical Medicine, 1990–1995; thereafter Environmental Health Group, EHG)
EW	Extension Worker
GARNET	Global Applied Research Network
IRC	International Water and Sanitation Centre, The Hague, The Netherlands
KWA	Kerala Water Authority, Kerala, India
LSH&TM	London School of Hygiene & Tropical Medicine
NGO	Non-Governmental Organization
ODA	Overseas Development Administration (UK Government)
ORS	Oral Rehydration Solution
PRA	Participatory Rural Appraisal
PROWWESS	Promotion of the Role of Women in Water and Environmental Sanitation Services (a UNDP/World Bank special programme)
RAP	Rapid Assessment/Appraisal Procedures
RWSG-EA	Regional Water and Sanitation Group—East Africa
SANPLAT	Sanitary platform (type of latrine)
SEU	Socioeconomic Unit (part of Kerala Water Authority, Kerala, India)

SHEWAS   Siaya Health Education, Water and Sanitation Project, Kenya

TBA   Traditional Birth Attendant

UNDP   United Nations Development Programme

UNICEF   United Nations International Children's Emergency Fund

VIP   Ventilated Improved Pit (type of latrine)

WAMMA   WaterAid, *Maji, Maendeleo, Afya* (a WaterAid-supported intersectoral water supply, sanitation and hygiene education project in Dodoma region, Tanzania)

WHO   World Health Organization

Glossary

The following is a set of definitions of technical terms used in this handbook:

Evaluation. Systematic assessment or appraisal of existing hygiene practices focusing on what they are and why they are practiced.

Method. Manner, technique of doing something, for instance, gathering information on existing hygiene practices.

Observer effect. The effect of being watched; changing one's behaviour as a result of being observed.

Sensitize. To arouse awareness, to make people aware of, or sensitive to, things they had not previously noticed.

Stakeholder. Interested party, someone with shared ownership of something of importance, for example, the findings of a hygiene evaluation study.

Tool. Instrument. For example, an informal interview schedule is a tool for collecting information, as is a questionnaire. A tool can be applied using a variety of methods or techniques.

Triangulation. Crosschecking of information by looking at its different sources, methods and tools of obtaining it, and/or its differing versions as held by different investigators.

Introduction

This handbook consists of practical guidelines for evaluating water- and sanitation-related hygiene practices. Hygiene practices are routine actions, commonly associated with cleanliness. *Evaluation* may refer to a systematic assessment carried out during the early stages of project planning, halfway through project implementation, or at the end of project activities. An evaluation of hygiene practices can be done for the purposes of project planning, monitoring, or final assessment of the project's impact.

Evaluation

- For planning intervention
- For monitoring implementation
- For assessing the impact of intervention

If the objective is to plan or to design effective interventions for hygiene improvements, this handbook can be used as part of the project *planning* activities. If your project is at the planning stage, and you wish to include in the project hygiene promotion, education, or communication, this handbook may help you to gather systematic baseline information, to interpret or understand it, and then apply it when *implementing* your project. If you are already implementing a hygiene promotion project and you want to see whether you are going in the right direction, or whether you need to change direction to achieve better results, you can use this handbook for *monitoring* purposes. If your project had already collected systematic information on hygiene practices at the beginning, identified those to be targeted for improvement, and worked to bring about change in hygiene practices over a period of time, then this handbook can help you to *measure change in hygiene practices* and thereby *assess the impact* of your project. This handbook can therefore be used for a variety of evaluation purposes depending on the project objectives that are to be met.

DIAGRAM 1
Contents of this Handbook

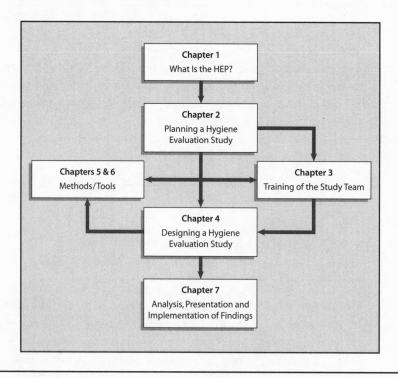

1

What Is the HEP?

■ *Why Assess Hygiene Practices?*

■ *Who Is This Handbook For?*

■ *Is This a Participatory Handbook?*

The Hygiene Evaluation Procedures (HEP) handbook was conceived of as a field companion to *Actions Speak: the study of hygiene behaviour in water and sanitation projects* (Boot and Cairncross, 1993), a resource book prepared primarily for project managers and decision-makers. In contrast, the HEP's main focus is on the practical concerns of field personnel in water supply, sanitation, and health/hygiene education projects who want to design and conduct their own evaluations of hygiene practices.

This handbook was developed through processes of consultation with a number of field-level project staff working in Eastern Africa (rural Kenya, Tanzania, and selected urban areas in Ethiopia). Each consultation process involved a hygiene evaluation study designed and conducted by project staff with coordination, training, and supervision support from researchers whose backgrounds include anthropology, community development, and public health. Practical insights gained from these studies reflect the needs and concerns of the primary intended users. The draft HEP was field tested in India and Afghanistan prior to peer review and finalization.

The emphasis of the HEP is on how to gather, review, and interpret qualitative information. In line with related manuals and handbooks designed to provide technical/methodological support to health practitioners (see, for instance, Simpson-Herbert, 1983; Scrimshaw and

Hurtado, 1987), the HEP handbook is designed to make qualitative research skills accessible to practitioners with little or no previous training in the social sciences. It is not for quantitative researchers who want to use statistical analysis. Qualitative information is gathered, analyzed, and interpreted differently from quantitative information, but this does not mean that the two types of information cannot be gathered and analyzed side-by-side to enable a fuller understanding of the issues under study.

The quality of information collected is critical in the systematic assessment of hygiene practices. A number of problems have been identified in relation to the quality of questionnaire-based data due to the limitations of the questionnaire as the sole instrument for information gathering (see Gill, 1993 for a concise analysis). The problems are more pronounced where sociocultural information is sought. However, qualitative information collected with the aim of designing good questionnaires for specific topics of enquiry can improve the effectiveness of questionnaires. This handbook was developed as a practical solution to the limitations of using a single method or instrument for information gathering, especially when trying to investigate sociocultural aspects of human behaviour that do not easily lend themselves to quantifiable measurement.

Like previous works on the subject of assessing hygiene practices, the HEP explores alternatives to the questionnaire-based survey design by examining other tools for the systematization of gathering chiefly qualitative information. We do not discourage you from using questionnaires. Many projects use and will continue to use questionnaire-based surveys on which to base their decisions. However, we advocate the use of trustworthy qualitative information with which to design your questionnaire, and the use of other tools to complement your questionnaire. The triangulation of sources and methods is advocated as the best way to obtain a complete set of information on the issues under study.

In order to emphasize *practicality*, we have included:

■ a variety of methods and tools from which you can choose and combine;

■ appraisals of individual methods and tools to help you select the most appropriate combination(s) of methods for your purposes;

■ examples from field experience including common mistakes and pitfalls to provide insight into what a hygiene evaluation study may involve.

Why Assess Hygiene Practices?

For a long time, project planners have appreciated the value of improving water supply and sanitation facilities. Improved facilities reduce contamination of drinking water and of the environment, and reduce diarrhoeal disease transmission and worm infestations. Even so, World Health Organization and World Bank statistics show that as many as three million children still die from intestinal infections every year, and a third of the world's population is still infected with parasites. The main reason for this is not that *too little* has been invested in technological improvement of facilities, but that the facilities are often inappropriate, unaffordable, or unacceptable to the intended users. All of these result in no use, limited use, or inappropriate use of facilities.

For example, pit latrines are widely promoted in both urban and rural regions in many parts of the world, in order to prevent faeces from contaminating the environment. However, having the facility does not in itself guarantee the isolation of faecal contamination. Even where pit latrines are in use, faecal contamination can get into drinking water and food and thereby into the mouth, or directly from fingers into the mouth. Various routes of transmission, such as fingers, flies, soil, and water, may require different barriers if the spread of contamination is to be stopped. This makes the prevention of diarrhoea and worm infections complex, as shown in Figure 1.

This diagram, often called the *F diagram*, clearly shows the different transmission routes whereby pathogens can get from the faeces of an infected person through *fluids* (mainly drinking water), *fields* (soil), *fingers*, and *food*. Some of the most effective primary and secondary (behavioural) barriers are indicated. You can see that there are at least nine barriers/facilities associated with hygiene practices. Clearly, numbers 1 and 2, pit latrines and Ventilated Improved Pit (VIP) latrines respectively, are very important physical barriers. If they are constructed and used properly, they can prevent faeces from contaminating water sources, soil, and food. The rest of the barriers relate to hygiene practices such as the protection of water sources (4) irrespective of the existence of latrines; hand-washing at critical times—after defecation, after cleaning children's bottoms, before handling food, and before eating and/or feeding (5); protection of food by safe storage (6); safe handling (7); protection of water in transit and in the home (8); and, washing raw foods before eating them (9).

Do improved hygiene practices really make a difference to health? Research shows that hygiene-related practices such as the safe disposal of

FIGURE 1
Faeco-Oral Routes of Disease Transmission

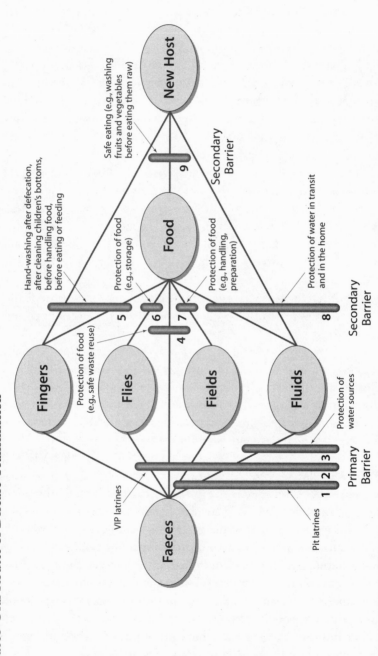

faeces and hand-washing after contact with faecal material can reduce the rates of intestinal infection considerably. Consider the following figures:

■ *Hand-washing* with soap and water can reduce diarrhoeal disease by 35% or more. Hand-washing can also help to reduce the prevalence of eye infections such as conjunctivitis and trachoma.

■ *Safe disposal of faeces* serves as a primary barrier to prevent faeces from contaminating the environment. It is particularly important to isolate the faeces of people with diarrhoea, most of whom are usually young children. Pit latrines, when used by adults and for the disposal of young children's stools, can reduce diarrhoea by 36% or more.

■ *Protection of water* from faecal contamination can also reduce diarrhoea, because some diarrhoeal infections are water-borne. Water quality in the home can be improved by using only a protected water source for drinking purposes; by keeping water storage vessels clean, covered, and out of the reach of young children and domestic animals; by boiling water where practical; or by putting water in clear plastic containers and exposing them to sunshine for several hours. In the special case of guinea worm, filtering with a cloth filter can provide complete protection. Improved water quality can be associated with up to a 20% reduction in diarrhoea. However, increased quantity of water used, which results from better access to water, can bring about still greater reductions.

However, much remains to be learned about the links between improved water supply and sanitation facilities, and well-designed and implemented health/hygiene promotion and health. What is clear is that good hygiene practices are necessary for maintaining good health.

Who is This Handbook For?

This handbook was developed primarily for field level personnel in water supply, sanitation, and hygiene education projects. These include water and/or sanitary engineers, public health technicians, community workers, health educators, communication specialists, health workers, and other public health practitioners as well as project planners, managers, and trainers. If you are one of these, and want to design your own assessment of hygiene practices in your project site, this handbook is for you. This handbook may also be useful to students and researchers in public health and other academic institutions interested in interdisciplinary enquiries into health behaviour.

Successful systematic investigations are seldom done by one person or with one perspective alone. The skills and experiences of engineers, health workers, and community development workers are all relevant when trying to investigate and analyze activities around water supply and sanitation. You will need to involve in your assessment your colleagues and other people who know and understand the local social and cultural norms. This handbook provides examples of a variety of tools designed to make the participation of local people in your assessment effective. Therefore it is also aimed, indirectly, at those whose hygiene practices are to be assessed.

Is This a Participatory Handbook?

One of the issues encountered during the development of this handbook was the question of whether or not outsiders (researchers and/or project staff) should do all the investigation and analysis in hygiene evaluation studies, without involving the people studied. No assessments of hygiene practices can be done by outsiders alone, without the participation of the people studied. The problem is that the term *participatory* is used widely to mean different things to different people. Researchers working in the fields of agriculture as well as water supply and sanitation projects have identified several uses of the term *participation* or *community participation*. White (1981) has identified ten and Pretty (1994) seven different types of participation. Box 1 provides an outline of three main types of participation.

BOX 1

Three Types of Participation (Adapted from Pretty, 1994)

Extractive
People participate by answering questions posed by researchers using questionnaire surveys or similar approaches. People do not have the opportunity to influence proceedings, as the findings of the research are neither shared nor checked for accuracy.

Consultative
People participate by being consulted, and external agents listen to views. These external agents define both problems and solutions, and may modify these in the light of people's responses. [Such a consultative process does not concede any share in decision-making, and professionals are under no obligation to adopt people's views.]

Interactive
People participate in joint analysis, which leads to action plans and the formation of new local institutions or the strengthening of existing ones. It tends to involve interdisciplinary methodologies that seek multiple perspectives and make use of systematic and structured learning processes. These groups take control over local decisions, and so people have a stake in maintaining structures or practices.

You must decide which of these types of participation coincide with your project's ethos and approach. The purpose of this handbook is not to prescribe any particular brand of participatory approach. Our aim is to show how combining methods and tools from *participatory* and *conventional*, or *nonparticipatory* ways of investigation can produce good quality information, and therefore a better understanding of the issues under investigation.

In conclusion, how participatory you may want to make your hygiene evaluation study may largely depend on your answers to the following two main questions:

- To what extent have local people been involved in the planning, design, and implementation of your project? For instance, if the provision of protected water sources and getting individual households to acquire latrines are part of your project activities, to what extent did you involve members of your target population in discussions of your project aims and objectives? To what extent have your project plans taken into account local needs, beliefs, and priorities?

- What institutional mechanisms are there to put the findings of your hygiene assessment to immediate use? For example, do you foresee the possibilities of changing the direction of project activities if that is what the findings of your assessment suggest? Who would take responsibility for any necessary changes to be put into effect and how?

2

Planning a Hygiene Evaluation Study

■ *What Am I Going to Investigate?*

■ *What Types of Information Will I Need?*

■ *Who Will Be Involved?*

■ *What Resources Will I Need?*

■ *When Should I Do a Hygiene Evaluation Study?*

You will need to plan your investigation in as much detail as possible. For example, you can start by asking what do I want to investigate? How much time and other resources do I have? Who is going to be involved? When? Answers to these questions, however sketchy and preliminary, will shape your plan of investigation.

What Am I Going to Investigate?

You may start by writing down the question(s) to be addressed. For example:

■ *What are the existing problems and priorities concerning sanitation and water supply in my project area?* This question will require you to make direct contact with the inhabitants of the area to engage them in *defining the problems* and ranking them according to importance/ priority. This is an effective way of involving local people in your *planning*. If improved water supply and/or sanitation facilities rate high in their list of priorities, then assessing existing water and sanitation-related practices will lead you to identify appropriate ways of meeting these priorities. The outcome of a hygiene evaluation study can be expected to provide baseline data which can form the foundation of a well-designed project.

If you are designing a hygiene evaluation study half-way through the implementation of project activities, the resulting information may enable you to *monitor* the progress of activities and either to continue with existing plans of action or to modify them as appropriate.

If the assessment of hygiene practices is being carried out at the end of project activities, the results may provide you with some indication of what has been achieved by the project, directly or indirectly. If the improvement of hygiene practices has been a project goal and baseline data had been previously collected, this assessment will enable you to measure change in hygiene practices by comparing your findings with the baseline data.

■ *Are the sanitation and water supply facilities promoted or provided by my project being used as intended? If not, why not?* Answers to these questions will help you find out how much progress has been made or whether a change of direction is needed in your project implementation. These questions can be posed whether or not appropriate use of facilities had been part of your project's original objectives.

■ *How successful has my project been in promoting improvement or change in hygiene practices?* This question can only be addressed successfully by a hygiene evaluation study if your project had collected information on existing hygiene practices before the start of its hygiene promotion, education, or communication activities. Otherwise, the outcome of a study using this handbook can only be used to describe the situation at the time of the study. You will not be able to measure behaviour change because you have no baseline data against which to measure change.

All of these questions are of a general nature and will need to be developed further into specific questions that apply to your particular setting.

What Types of Information Will I Need?

In order to assess hygiene practices and to understand why they occur in the way they do, you will need to gather diverse types of information. Some of these may already exist in your project files and/or other written documents, while others will need to be collected during your hygiene evaluation study.

The Physical Environment

Climate, terrain, soil type, and availability of water may all influence hygiene practices. For example, people are not likely to use water for washing or bathing frequently if there is very little water available near them and if they have to walk long distances to fetch water for everyday use. Similarly, pastoralist communities who live in very arid regions and move periodically from one area to another are not likely to be concerned about building sanitary facilities.

Different sources may be available for you to use to research this information. There may be written records with detailed descriptions of the area, perhaps with historical perspectives. Ministries of Agriculture, Forestry, and/or Natural Resources may have records you can consult: usually, their annual reports provide some maps and photographs.

However, one of the best ways to collect relevant information on the physical environment is to go out and see, smell, touch, and feel the place of interest for yourself. Visits to existing water sources in and outside villages and familiarity with different parts of villages, districts, and regions around you are necessary if you want to learn about the physical conditions and features of your project site. Try to visit the study site when you start planning, so that you can plan your activities with the particular place in mind. You learn more by visiting villages yourself (and preferably staying in them for more than a day at a time), than by learning about them secondhand. Repeat visits at different times of the year are often necessary to appreciate seasonal variations in climate, water availability, accessibility of villages, agricultural workload of the inhabitants, and so on. Repeat visits also give you the chance to build up friendships with the inhabitants, so you can learn more from them as well as from your own observations.

The Population

Before meeting people in your study site, try to find out as much as possible about them. You (and your study team) need to ask yourselves the questions in Box 2.

Once you have answered these questions, you will be able to describe the *population* and the *community*. Be clear though, to whom you are referring when you use these terms. A few definitions may be useful:

Population. A defined group of people. The population of a country refers to all people in the country; the population of a village refers to all people in the village.

BOX 2

Preparing for the Study

■ How much do I know about the people served by my project?

■ Which language(s) do they speak?

■ Do I speak the local language(s)?

■ If not, which language am I going to use for communicating with local people?

■ Am I going to use interpreters? If so, who?

■ Which ethnic groups are represented?

■ Which religious affiliations exist?

■ Does my project have direct contact with ordinary people as opposed to community leaders and administrators or health workers only?

■ Have I visited and made contact with people in their day-to-day activities?

■ How much do I know about the local subsistence activities?

■ Have I been to the market place(s)?

■ Have I visited local people in their homes?

Study Population. This refers to all people you include in the study or evaluation. It is up to you to define them. The *study population* may be a sample of the total population of a given area.

Village. This term may refer to an administrative area and a geographic area (a group of houses close together), or it may be used only to refer to the administrative area including outlying land. When we talk about villages, however, we usually refer to a number of houses positioned closely together, which share some public facilities—a meeting place or common land, a well, a place of worship such as a mosque, temple, church, or schoolhouse.

Community. A community is a group of people with a shared identity and common interests. People may share a common interest because of their residence, or because of ethnic, language, religious, or other ties.

Family. This term is used to indicate that a group of people are related to each other by blood or by marriage. Not all members of a family will constitute a household, and not all householders may be related or part of a family.

Household. A household is conventionally defined as a group of people who share a single cooking pot. It can include nuclear families (husband, wife, and children only), extended families (additional family members, often grandparents as well), households with more than one wife, and households where not all members are related. In general, households include people usually related, who live under one roof, and share certain economic resources.

Note that all of these terms need to be defined. The term *community*, for example, seldom refers to a homogeneous group of people. A village community is usually made up of subgroups such as elders, leaders, men, women, and children, and poor and wealthy family groups who may belong to different clans or ethnic groups. The village community may be made up of people who belong to the same language or ethnic group but do not necessarily share the same views or beliefs. People from two different ethnic or language groups in the same area, even in the same village, may be regarded as—and much more importantly, they may regard themselves as—belonging to one community sometimes, and two communities on other occasions.

You cannot assume that these groups share the same views or have the same interests. You need to be sensitive to any conflicting interests within your study population. Men and women may represent significantly different interests. There may be differences even within these two gender groups. Some may be traditional while others are modernist. Some may be conformists while others are rebels.

In urban areas, people may consider themselves to be part of one or more interest groups, types of *community* that do not necessarily share the same ethnic, linguistic, cultural, or religious affiliations, but have similarly felt or expressed needs and concerns. If you use the term community, make sure you understand what it stands for, and define it carefully.

Gender

You need to collect and interpret information that is *gender-specific*. In other words, you should be able to come up with information that is specific to men, information that is specific to women, and information that is common to both men and women. Many hygiene-related activities have gender-specific roles and values associated with them. You need to ask women about their activities. Do not rely on men telling you what women do, or why they do it. Similarly, do not rely on women to describe men's activities.

For example, women and young children are often solely responsible for fetching water, and men's accounts of accessibility and use of water may be very different from women's. Women are also the first health and hygiene educators in the home. Sanitation and hygiene-related habits are inculcated at a very early age when toilet training and personal cleanliness are strongly influenced by the mother's teaching and practice.

Gender-specific roles may influence the adoption of sanitation facilities. In many cultures, the construction of pit latrines is seen as a man's job while the task of cleaning them is be a woman's. In rural western Kenya, women-headed households may face difficulties with latrine construction and repair, because it is not acceptable for a woman to dig a pit latrine or to repair a latrine with a leaking roof.

Hygiene Practices and Health

In order to identify practices that pose health hazards, you will need to find out which water and sanitation-related diseases are prevalent in the project site. This can be done by consulting the local dispensary, clinic, or hospital personnel, and their records. There may also be other institutions including your own project, which may have conducted health surveys or compiled records.

More importantly, you will need to find out what local people do about health-related problems. There may be documentary sources of information on existing health practices, including traditional practices, but there may still be more for you to find out. Understanding what the local population perceive to be *good* practices and *bad* ones (those that promote health and those that do not) and why, is an important contribution that your evaluation can make towards the design of an effective health or hygiene promotion intervention. You may be able to provide information on which good hygiene practices to encourage and which bad or harmful ones to try to discourage in acceptable ways.

Your study plan should include some detail of whether the different types of information will be qualitative, quantitative, or a combination of both. The units of analysis used and the sampling strategies applied will depend on the type of information gathered in terms of the qualitative-quantitative mix. As mentioned in the introduction, the emphasis of this handbook is on the depth or richness of information on hygiene practices that can be gathered through qualitative methods, and that can help project personnel better understand the cultural and social context in which they work. Whether or not the study is designed to include quantitative data also will depend on the resources available. The two approaches can be adopted side by side to address questions of breadth and depth at the same time. A qualitative study ideally *always* precedes the quantitative investigation, especially for baseline evaluation purposes. However, qualitative research can also be preceded by a quantitative survey, which might identify certain issues to be followed up, using qualitative methods, for clarification and further detail.

Who Will Be Involved?

A hygiene evaluation study will involve different people and will concern them in different ways. Identify the main stakeholders: those who are going to be involved in and ultimately affected by it—the *primary stakeholders*, and those who are going to have some intermediary role, the *secondary stakeholders* (see ODA, 1995).

Ethical Issues

Before you set out to conduct your hygiene evaluation study, you must get the consent of your study participants. This may include written consent, although this may not be possible if the participants are illiterate or if they regard forms and the provision of their names and/or signatures as intrusive or threatening. The following guideline may be helpful to gain informed consent:

- Explain the purpose of your study to official representatives of your study population(s) as well as to community leaders. These may include elders, religious leaders, and other senior men and women who have socially influential roles in the locality.

- Explain the purpose of the study to your informants (study participants) as well. Assure them that you are not going to use the information they provide against them, and keep your promise. Assure them, too, that you will preserve the anonymity of individual study participants when reporting results of your investigation. People rarely wish to be publicly identified with sensitive information obtained during a study. If you do wish to quote someone, or to present information that could lead to a participant being identified, you should gain his or her permission to do so.

- Strive to make the results of your investigation available to local institutions, both formal and informal, such as government departments and village committees, in ways they can use. Giving feedback of your study findings to participants will increase the credibility of the findings, as they will check them for accuracy. It will also enhance your project's relationship with the target populations.

Ownership of Information

Who will own the data? This question is best addressed before data collection and analysis begin. Where collaborative arrangements have been made at the outset of the study, each party must have a clear understanding as to who will need access to the information (or parts of it) and who is to provide that access. The question of who *owns* the data is often difficult to answer because various stakeholders may want to assume direct or indirect entitlement to be custodians of information. Among the most common stakeholders are:

■ the external agency who financed the study;

■ the project manager who needs to use the data to monitor progress and account to funding bodies, make decisions about further action, and so on;

■ the participants who spent their time and energy cooperating with the study team in providing, analysing, and interpreting the data;

■ those who conducted the study, who wish to make parts of their report available to others (e.g., by publishing).

Problems can arise if one of these stakeholders claims exclusive ownership of the data at the end of the study. For this reason, you must agree on a fair and workable arrangement at the outset.

Who Will Be in the Study Team?

Most projects include staff of varied personal as well as professional skills, and abilities. You will need to include the range of skills available and allocate tasks appropriately. For example, a member of staff with graduate level qualification (diploma or certificate in public health, sanitary engineering, social development or health work) may be the person to take responsibility for documentation of results and report writing. Another member with highly developed communication skills may be allocated tasks of facilitating group discussions, interviewing, or organizing the activities of the team.

Skills

List individual skills and capabilities in your project. A good study team may include people with the following qualities:

- At least one or two persons who belong to the local population or culture and are good communicators. Members of study populations, such as village health workers, traditional birth attendants, water pump attendants, and women's group leaders may be recruited and trained.

- At least two or three persons (project staff) who have good writing skills and can commit themselves to the study from start to finish.

- Other project staff who are senior may already have experience working with the project. Such persons are often invaluable when it comes to translating the study findings into an action plan. Ideally, they should be included in the study team in the preplanning stage and also, if possible, in at least some of the investigation and analysis sessions.

Do not include in your study team:

- Persons who are unwilling or unable to assume the role of a learner in relation to the study population. A person who has difficulties in showing respect to local people and engaging with them on an equal footing may be more of a liability than an asset to your team.

- Persons who are unable or unwilling to stay in poorer areas than they normally live in. For example, the work required to carry out your hygiene evaluation study may require you to spend a lot of time in the poorest parts of a town or in rural areas where eating and sleeping arrangements may be very rudimentary.

Each member of the study team will need to be:

- interested in learning about how to assess hygiene practices in their cultural, socioeconomic, and physical context;

- willing and able to learn and to adopt new skills and attitudes (this may involve unlearning old ones) for effective communication with members of the population(s) under study;

- prepared to initiate and maintain a team spirit with other members of the team/colleagues.

Conflict

If there is conflict in the study population, try to avoid including, in the study team, persons who are affiliated with only one side of the conflict.

Make sure you include only neutral persons such as teachers, health workers, or extension workers who do not belong to any one group, but live in the locality, or include at least one representative of each of the conflicting groups.

It is not usually a good idea to work closely with political leaders, or to have someone with political connections in your study team, as this can affect how people perceive you, and bias your findings. However, you may wish to include people with political connections in your discussions and interviews during the investigation and analyses. Such people may include political leaders as well as members of their families. Conduct a *Stakeholder Analysis* to enable you to make pragmatic decisions (see Box 3 for guidance on how to do a Stakeholder Analysis).

Language

It is essential to have in your study team, persons who are native speakers of the local language(s), as this improves the quality of information gathered. If necessary, other members of the team who are fluent in English can translate for them when reviewing and documenting their information.

What Resources Will I Need?

Write down the amount of resources available to you for use in a hygiene evaluation study. Remember that *resources* include:

- People
- Time
- Space
- Money

BOX 3
How to Do a Stakeholder Analysis (Adapted from ODA, 1995)

There are several steps to doing a Stakeholder Analysis:

- Draw up a "stakeholder table." To do this you need to identify and list all potential stakeholders; identify their interests (overt and hidden) in relation to your study aims and objectives; and determine whether the impact of your study on each of these interests is likely to be positive, negative or unknown.

- Determine each stakeholder's possible role in making use of the study findings and their relative power to act/influence.

- Identify risks and assumptions which will affect the study design and success.

It may be that your project has budgeted some money for an evaluation. Find out how much *time* can be budgeted and *who* can be assigned to carry out the evaluation. When considering time and human resources, do not restrict your vision to your collaborators or fellow project staff only. Think about ways to involve the people who are going to supply the information you require for the study. You will need to carry out a preplanning piece of investigation to find out *who* your study populations are, what activity patterns they follow by season, income level, or social status, *when* might be a good time for them to be involved in your study, and *what* they might expect to get out of it. You will need to consider all of these before you decide how you are going to use your resources.

The following are some of the items of expenditure that should be included in your budget:

■ *Training* of the study team. This may require hiring a specially designated venue such as a hotel, conference centre, or residential school where the initial training of the study team can be carried out.

■ *Transportation* (vehicle maintenance and fuel). If your project owns vehicle(s), you will need to make prior arrangements to make sure that the study team can travel freely during the conduct of fieldwork.

■ *Subsistence* in the study site. Food, drink and accommodation for the study team, including the driver(s), should be included in the budget, to avoid unnecessary discomfort or inconvenience during the study period.

■ *Remuneration* for project staff who are going to put in extra hours of work during the study. Project staff will be required to work overtime and to spend time away from their families while conducting the study. This may incur extra expenses particularly for mothers of young children. In addition, many people in poor countries survive by holding a second job, and if they are working away from home, they will not be able to do this. The study coordinator should agree to reasonable payments in cash or in kind, as appropriate.

■ *Allocate some space* to the study team, if possible a room to use for meetings, preparation of materials, further training and documentation, as well as for data management, analysis, and report writing. Show all members of your team your appreciation at the end of the study by giving them something. This could be in cash or kind, depending on what is appropriate to the particular project and in the local cultural context.

When Should I Do a Hygiene Evaluation Study?

The timing of your study will depend on your answers to the following questions:

■ Do your project objectives include improvements in hygiene practices? If not, then the results of your investigation will not be linked to project objectives, but may be used in redirecting your project goals. If your project is about to come to an end, the main reason for conducting a hygiene evaluation study may be to gain a detailed insight into existing hygiene practices for the record, or possibly to consider in future interventions. If your project is a pilot project, then your study may influence future projects.

■ Which methods has your project already applied for monitoring its effectiveness? Are there many records you need to gather, review, and digest before you set out on this study? How much time will that require?

■ Do you know when the best times are for you and your colleagues to work on the project? Do you have financial deadlines coming up soon? If the end of a project financial year is imminent, there may be

---

BOX 4

Financial Arrangements for the Study Team

In one study, project staff were paid weekly cash allowances to cover subsistence (food and drink). Transportation costs (vehicle, maintenance, fuel) were handled separately. The (external) study coordinator provided materials (paper, flip charts, notebooks, pens, etc.). At the end of the study, the team took tea, sugar, bread, and biscuits to the villages where they had worked to share with some of the study participants (those present). The village health workers who acted as support members of the study team were rewarded for their efforts in kind (items of local clothing were purchased for them). Project staff were treated to an end-of-study celebration meal and given token rewards for their efforts. This reinforced the sense of team spirit and shared ownership of the study results.

In another study, community members of the study team were given rewards in kind— project staff shared their food and drink with them. At the end of the study, the key collaborators (all women) were each given a new garment in recognition of their contribution to the study. The project staff were paid allowances in cash to cover their field expenses. Camping gear was provided by the project (tents, camp beds, blankets, water containers, plastic plates, cups and cutlery, a solar lantern, kerosene lanterns, and small torches.) Tents were not used for security reasons, but the rest of the camping equipment was used in village owned buildings, such as meeting rooms and school rooms, where the study team was allowed to stay.

funds left over that need to be spent quickly. However, will you and your colleagues have the time to implement a good hygiene evaluation study? Remember that money is only part of what is needed. What about your collaborators, including government ministries, agencies, and/or trainers? Will your timing easily correspond with theirs?

- Do you know whether and when members of your study population are likely to be willing and interested in participating in your investigation? For example, if they live in a rural area, they will be especially busy at harvest time. They may have been involved in several other studies, and be reluctant to participate without considerable consideration and negotiation. You may also need to allow extra time if climatic conditions make travelling difficult at certain times of year or if climatic conditions will affect study results. For example, heavy rain and prolonged drought both have extreme effects on water and sanitation.

3

Training the Study Team

■ *Sensitizing the Study Team*

■ *Transferring Technical Know-How*

■ *Management, Review, and Analysis of Information*

■ *Developing Working Hypotheses*

■ *Outlining the Study Design*

■ *What Resources Are Needed?*

■ *How Much Time Should Be Allowed for Training?*

Once you have established your study team, you will need to assign a suitably experienced applied anthropologist or related *social scientist*, a trainer who can guide and supervise the study team during planning, designing, and conducting the study. Some projects already have highly trained staff. Training may be given periodically by external or in-house trainer(s). Other projects may have less trained and/or skilled personnel. This chapter provides some guidelines for the trainer who must take into account existing skills when planning and conducting initial as well as on-the-job training.

The purpose of training is threefold:

■ to prepare and sensitize the study team for the disciplined task of qualitative investigation of the sociocultural determinants of hygiene practices;

- to equip the team with the technical knowledge and skills required to carry out such an investigation;

- to involve the study team in designing the study with a view to conducting it themselves.

These three are equally important purposes of training because the attitude and behaviour of the study team can influence the quality of information obtained, as much as the team's skills of investigation and analysis can. In addition, it is easier for the study team to conduct a study designed with the help of team participation than it is to carry out a study that has been designed by one or more individuals prior to the team's engagement.

Sensitizing the Study Team

To sensitize means "to make sensitive" and is a term widely used in *participatory* research as well as in anthropological circles where the ability to recognize local/lay knowledge is highly appreciated. The term is less known in circles that uphold the premise that knowledge comes from the academic and/or technical "expert" and should be transmitted to the "ignorant" lay or local person.

Investigating hygiene practices systematically is not something that comes naturally to the average water supply and sanitation project worker, particularly if his/her training background and/or experience does not include qualitative investigations. For example, the average water or sanitary technician concentrates on pumps and pipes and does not see the need to find out what the users of those pumps and pipes are doing, what they have to say, and why.

It is important for each member of the study team to be trained to be inquisitive and not assume that she/he knows what is going on in the locality. It is very important to adopt a *learner's* attitude, however difficult that might first appear to someone whose job it has been to *teach the people*.

Encourage the study team to discuss the following ways of establishing rapport with the study population, and to identify the most relevant points for their own setting. People will react towards members of the study team according to their gender, ethnicity, age, style of dress and speech, and how they present themselves. Individually and as a team, investigators should aim to minimize status differences so that people can feel comfortable with them. This will bring about cooperation and minimize the "observer effect," where people act or say things that are not usual because of the presence of strangers. It will also help to minimize possible bias as a result of the observer effect.

Suggested ways of establishing rapport include:

■ *Appearance.* This is very important. For example, when working in a rural community, try to identify with local people and minimize the gaps that exist by wearing simple clothes and using simple language. The reverse may be necessary when talking to professionals or top level personnel, you would dress to suit the occasion, but without drawing unnecessary attention to yourself.

■ *Greeting.* This is more effective in the local language, especially when in rural settings. If you are not a speaker of the native language, it is helpful to learn at least a few basic words to demonstrate your interest.

■ *Introduction.* Introduce yourself and ask the person you are addressing to introduce herself or himself, in a locally acceptable manner. This is particularly important in the case of interviews. In group discussions, each participant should be invited to introduce themselves. This will help to assure study participants that investigators are genuinely interested in learning about them.

■ *Terms of address.* When asking questions, use the respondent's name, with the appropriate title, whenever applicable. This helps information gathering (particularly interviews) to remain informal or conversational rather than formal or interrogative. The person being asked questions should not feel that they are on trial or being given a test about what they know.

■ *Establish confidence* by stressing to the study participants that you are interested in her/his/their opinions, knowledge and beliefs. In the context of individual interviews or group discussions, make it clear that your intention is to *learn* and not to judge.

■ *Establish confidentiality* by assuring the study participants that your conversations or interviews will not be repeated to others and that when you write a report, they will not be identified by name.

Once established, good rapport with the study population can be maintained by observing certain universal rules of courtesy which include the following:

■ *Privacy.* Investigators should be very careful about intruding in people's privacy. Private and sensitive questions such as asking to see people's latrines can cause embarrassment; so might asking about income.

However, this can be minimized if the study team ensures that the participants are well-informed about the investigators' motives and interests. If people understand why you are asking them such questions, they are more likely to cooperate with you.

■ *Timing*. Visits to people's homes and the timing of group discussion meetings should take into account local patterns of activities. For example, investigators should avoid arriving for interviews at meal times. Make sure that you consult people before setting the dates and time for group meetings. You will need to be flexible enough to allow for possible rescheduling of activities during local holy days, market days, and other less predictable events such as, for instance, funerals.

■ *Feedback*. Presenting the findings to the study population(s) informs those who participated in your study, and provides them with the opportunity to comment on your conclusions, to confirm your analysis, to correct any misconceptions, and perhaps also to provide additional information. Feedback helps people to increase awareness of their own hygiene practices, and to appreciate the reasons for your project's interventions. Seeing that you have taken the trouble to let your informants see the results of their cooperation, using flip-charts or summary sheets, may help them to remain interested and cooperative during the study period and beyond.

Transferring Technical Know-How

Training should enable the study team to learn new skills and/or improve old skills in how to use qualitative methods of investigation and analysis. It is difficult to generalize on the skills and qualifications that project staff are expected to have, as this varies greatly from one project to another. It may be that some projects have employees with social science training and/or experience, but this is not common. Many project staff such as sanitary/water engineers, public health technicians, and health/hygiene education specialists will have considerable knowledge about environmental, microbiological, and epidemiological aspects of water supply and sanitation interventions. Those who work on the social development and educational side of the project may know more about the social, cultural, and behavioural aspects.

It is important to assess existing skills and identify areas where training and supervision should concentrate. The trainer should find out what members of the study team have already done and build on their knowledge and skills as much as possible, rather than introduce a completely new set of skills which will require more time to master.

The social scientific skills required to systematically assess hygiene practices and related issues are best learned using a combination of both theoretical and practical training methods. On the theoretical front, the trainer may give informal talks or seminars and point out key references or resource materials for the study team to read. A study resource stock-pile consisting of essential reading and/or reference materials may include some of those listed in the *Selected Reading* list at the end of this hand-book. During the initial training, encourage each member of the study team to read at least one item and to share their thoughts on it with the group. This will facilitate relatively quick assimilation of information and stimulate discussion of new ideas. On the practical front, the focus should be on activities that enhance the team's investigative and analytical skills.

The following suggestions might be included in classroom and field training sessions. The methods and tools for assessing hygiene practices described in this handbook require three main skill categories: observation, interviewing, and facilitating, moderating, or leading group discussions. Each category is discussed with reference to the particular method/tool that requires each skill.

Observation Skills

The term observation relates not only to looking or the sense of sight, but also to the senses of touch, feel, and smell. However, having functioning senses does not automatically make a person a skilled observer. Training is required in order to know what to look for, to sharpen one's senses and also to record or document one's observations. Observers need to learn how to:

■ write systematic detailed descriptions of what is observed;

■ separate relevant detail from trivia without being overwhelmed by the amount of trivia.

It is often difficult to train people to be good observers because, as Patton put it, "...so many people think that they are 'natural' observers and therefore have very little to learn. Training to become a skilled observer is a no less rigorous process than the training necessary to become a skilled statistician. People don't 'naturally' know statistics—and people don't 'naturally' know how to do systematic research observations. Both require training, practice and preparation." (Patton, 1990:201).

Conducting observations can demand considerable energy and concentration. The observer has to switch on her or his concentration to
awaken eyes, ears, taste, touch, and smell mechanisms. You cannot expect members of the study team to conduct systematic observations spon-
taneously without the training and mental preparation required. Skilled
observers can improve the accuracy and trustworthiness of observation
data through intensive training and rigorous preparation.

However, it is important to note that even skilled and well-trained
observers can bring in their own biases to the information. This may be
because of the observer effect, behaving differently due to the presence of
an observer. It may also be due to the inherent limitations of information
derived from observation only, and not from direct experience.

For example, a mother may wash her hands thoroughly after dispos-
ing of her baby's stools during the observer's visit because she wants to
give a good impression of herself. When the observer is not around, she
might just wipe her hands on her dress or apron or *sari,* and continue
with what she was doing before the baby defecated, and not worry about
washing her hands. This shows that the observer effect can produce
biased information. Similarly, an observer may notice that a woman
collecting water from the well has covered her water pot with leaves
before putting it on her head to take home. This observer may not be
familiar with this practice (commonly done in several parts of Africa to
prevent water from spilling while the woman carries it to her home) and
may interpret it as an imprudent (unnecessarily contaminating) practice
without asking the woman why she had done it.

For this reason, participant observation has in the past been seen as
the best method, if not the only method to obtain indepth information
on the issue under study. However, the term participant observation is an
umbrella term that includes observation, interview, and discussion. The
use of a combination of methods is certainly the way to minimize bias.
The observer's ultimate goal is to be able to understand and explain
observed phenomena as accurately as possible, but absolute accuracy may
not be achievable.

Observations can vary according to focus, duration, the role adopted
by the observer, and the way the observer's role is portrayed to the study
population (see Box 5). Trainees should be encouraged to:

- suggest whether they would envisage assuming the role of full participant observers, partial participant observers, or onlookers from outside, and state the reasons why with reference to their particular setting;

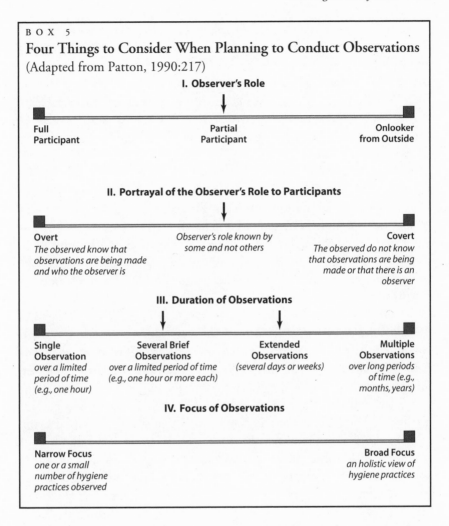

BOX 5

Four Things to Consider When Planning to Conduct Observations
(Adapted from Patton, 1990:217)

I. Observer's Role

| Full Participant | Partial Participant | Onlooker from Outside |

II. Portrayal of the Observer's Role to Participants

| Overt | Observer's role known by some and not others | Covert |
| The observed know that observations are being made and who the observer is | | The observed do not know that observations are being made or that there is an observer |

III. Duration of Observations

| Single Observation | Several Brief Observations | Extended Observations | Multiple Observations |
| over a limited period of time (e.g., one hour) | over a limited period of time (e.g., one hour or more each) | (several days or weeks) | over long periods of time (e.g., months, years) |

IV. Focus of Observations

| Narrow Focus | Broad Focus |
| one or a small number of hygiene practices observed | an holistic view of hygiene practices |

- discuss how observations would best be conducted in the study site(s) (whether observers should let the observed know what they are doing or keep it to themselves, and why);

- suggest what the duration of observations should be, and why;

- discuss whether the focus of observations will be broad or narrow, and why.

This will allow trainees to think about the use of observation methods analytically. Once developed, the techniques of observation can be used as integral parts of almost all the methods and tools described in Chapters

5 and 6. Direct observation is particularly an important part of conducting *healthwalk* and *semi-structured interviews,* but it is also built into the methods and tools that involve group discussion, because the interaction between participants of a group discussion is observed and noted as a matter of course in order to put in context the information gathered from that group. *Structured observations* carried out during home visits can provide vital information to help interpret data gathered by interviews conducted simultaneously.

Trainees may be given relatively short observations to conduct around the training place. For example, a healthwalk may be conducted in an afternoon for initial training purposes. First, describe in detail to participants what the healthwalk entails, and how it helps to orient the investigator to the study area. Trainees can be asked to conduct a healthwalk in the local area. This may involve a walk through the suburb surrounding the training site, or walk through a local market, or the neighbourhood of the project offices.

Trainees can be allowed up to an hour for the healthwalk, taking brief notes in a small note book. They should then return to the class/seminar room to write up more detailed notes and report to the group what they observed individually. Attention should be drawn to the variety of notes, differences in observation details, and systematic biases. For example, some people will routinely observe structures but not people; others may observe activities but not the circumstances in which activities take place, and so on.

Structured observations may be made using a checklist or tally sheet, if the items to be observed are precoded, or observations may be made systematically for the purposes of continuous monitoring and assessments of time-allocation for specific activities (see Bentley et al., 1994, for more examples).

Ask trainees to develop a checklist of things to observe in a given area. They can then make systematic observations using the checklist. They should also take notes of things not included in their checklist, or in relation to the items already included in the checklist, and later write these up. The notes might include details regarding participants, the nature of activities, and the time taken. Allow plenty of time for them to discuss their observations and the difficulties they faced.

As a result of the observation training exercises, participants' skills in observing activities, taking good notes, and awareness of observer bias should be improved. It should be emphasized that the aim is to document observed information and not to interpret or judge it on its own. Observation notes should give no indication of beliefs or attitudes of the people observed. These should be recorded separately. For example on the basis of observation alone, the study team should not conclude that women do not appreciate the advantage of a protected water source over an unprotected one. Discussions with women often reveal that water from a specific source is put to a specific use on the basis of rational decision-making processes.

Preparation and Pretesting of Observation Schedules

The preparation of a spot-check observation schedule (checklist) involves discussions of a draft checklist by the study team, translation into the local language(s), and back-translating from the local language into English in order to check the accuracy of meaning conveyed by translations. Trainees should spend some time reviewing the examples of structured (spot-check) observation schedules included in Chapters 5 and 6, and modifying them for use in their own study site(s).

Interviewing Skills

The two main skills required for successful interviewing are:

■ an ability to establish rapport with the interviewee, and

■ keen listening.

There are several exercises, role plays, and games that can be used to improve interviewing techniques, particularly in the areas of probing, listening, observing non-verbal cues, and recalling the content of interviews. These include:

Class Introductions

At the beginning of the training period, you can develop people's interviewing skills and establish rapport among the study team by asking them to form pairs, preferably with people they do not know well. The pair must interview each other about their life and their work sufficiently well in order to introduce each other to the group. Allow about twenty minutes for the interviews and then give each person two minutes to introduce the person interviewed.

Genealogical Exercises

Collecting a genealogy (a family history) is a good way to develop very focused interviewing skills. Again, get participants to form pairs—but different pairs from those of the preceding exercise. Get each to interview the other about family relationships, starting with the person being interviewed. In order to build up your picture of the family (or draw the family tree), you need to ask them about parents, siblings, sibling marriages, their own marriage, children, relatives of parents, and so on. Have all trainees discuss each of these in turn. Then ask each group member to take their own genealogy, and to draw a line around the people they live with, or those who live in the same village, town, or part of town. This can also be an effective way to introduce a discussion on defining units of analysis such as *family, household, homestead, community,* and so on.

Three-Way Interview Exercises

Ask trainees to form groups of three. Each person will in turn take on all three roles: the interviewer, the interviewee, and the observer. Choose any topic as the subject matter of the interview. The observer's role is to watch the interactions, observe possible leading questions or biases, monitor the use of prompts and probes, and note any areas overlooked by the interviewer. How well does the interviewee respond to this interviewer? After a set period of time, the three change roles, until all have had an opportunity to interview, be interviewed, and observe an interview. Ensure that there is plenty of time at the end to allow discussion of the interviews: everyone will have comments that relate to all of the roles they played, and they will learn further from listening to the feedback of others.

Saboteur

This is a game for trainees to identify ways of dealing with interruptions or break-up of communication that can happen during interviews. Trainees should again form groups of three, each taking the role of interviewer, informant/interviewee, and saboteur. The role of the saboteur, someone who engages in sabotaging the interview, can be illustrated using examples of interviewing a mother when the child(ren), the husband or a visitor is interfering in the conversation, without using violence. Examples of sabotage include interruptions, rude behaviour, such as staring, taking over the interview, and answering instead of the respondent, sitting in silence, and making noise. Each participant should have a chance to play each of the three roles and then to discuss the type of sabotage and possible ways to deal with it.

Among the ways to deal with sabotage are to:

- ignore the interruption;
- acknowledge it and deal with it immediately;
- acknowledge it and postpone dealing with it;

■ ask others for help or guidance;

■ involve the saboteur in the conversation;

■ stop the interview.

Once the trainees have played saboteur, you may find that they will keep identifying saboteurs in non-interview settings as well, for example, those who interrupt meetings and group discussions. The same principles can be applied to deal with saboteurs effectively. This game is fun to play and can help to maintain the study team's sense of humour, particularly if faced with unpleasant or unacceptable interruptions.

All of the above exercises should help the trainer(s) identify the best interviewers in the study team. These individuals can proceed to study the example of a semi-structured interview schedule included in Chapter 6. They should review and, if necessary, modify it to suit the specific objectives of the study. Encourage interviewers to be flexible when using preset question lines. The order in which questions are asked does not matter as much as the need to maintain an uninterrupted conversation with the interviewee. The order of questions should follow logically from the interviewee's responses. For example, questions about water use can be asked first if the informant's response to the first question has mentioned water use and not latrine use.

Group Discussion Moderating/Facilitating Skills

Many of the methods/tools described in this handbook involve group discussions that require skilled facilitators/moderators. Decisions about what methods/tools to try out during the training and which ones to prepare and use in the actual study should be based upon the study objectives, the capacity of the study team, and availability of time and material resources. Avoid choosing methods and tools just because they are part of the current fad in development and/or evaluation, without assessing their appropriateness to your study.

The trainer(s) may demonstrate how to facilitate *mapping* by getting participants to make a map of their town showing their project office, the local clinic or hospital, the departments of health, social development, water resources, education, and so on. If the group is large, you can divide the participants into two groups and get the second group to draw a detailed map of their project site. The role of facilitator and note-taker(s) may be played by the trainer(s) or by designated trainees. Allow about an hour for this exercise and discuss the outcome, highlighting areas of difficulty.

Similarly, a *historyline* (see Chapter 5) can be conducted among the trainees. Encourage the more senior/experienced members of the study team to recount the history of the project, agency, or department since its inception, or as early as they can remember. Get them to mark important events and key personalities on the historyline and elaborate on their significance. About forty minutes may be allowed for this exercise including the discussion of issues raised.

Seasonal calendars (see Chapter 5) can also be conducted to find out about the activities of project staff during the different seasons. This exercise may be used to find out the best time to conduct a hygiene evaluation, from the point of view of project staff. You can then get the project staff to conduct the same exercise during a visit to a nearby area to find out what local residents' schedules look like.

Three-pile sorting and/or gender roles/tasks analysis can also be tried if you already have the materials, or can prepare them relatively easily.

Focus group discussions may be tried by getting all trainees to participate in at least one focus group discussion on a topic of interest to them all. For example, "difficulties faced in doing field work" could serve as a good discussion topic. The results of such a discussion could also help the trainer to identify areas where on-the-job training should focus. Use Part II of the Focus Group Manual (Dawson, Manderson, and Tallo, 1993), which is wholly dedicated to the training of project staff on the use of focus group discussions. This includes plenty of examples of how to develop question lines, the use of probing and prompting techniques, note-taking and analysis of findings.

In the development and testing of this handbook, we have used a modified version of focus group discussions in which pictures are employed to introduce and stimulate discussion on sensitive topics (see Chapter 6). A point worth emphasizing is that the purpose of focus group discussions is to encourage participants to discuss the topic among themselves and is *not* to get them to respond to the moderator's questions one by one. This is a very common mistake where focus group discussions are said to have taken place when in actual fact they were group interviews.

The following exercises may be useful:

■ The trainees should develop some question-lines for the moderator/facilitator to use in the focus group. Stress that the question-lines should be much more general than an interview schedule—it should provide an outline only of the topics on which questions are to be asked.

■ Get members of the group to take turns moderating or facilitating the group discussion on a selected topic. Choose a few controversial topics in order to make the discussion stimulating, and take an extreme role yourself if people assume a common line and reach consensus too quickly. Alternatively, give participants particular roles to play (such as an extremist, a conformist, a rebel, a modernist, and so on) and have them act out their roles during the group discussion.

Interviewing and group discussion exercises can be continued for a couple of days until the trainer(s) are satisfied with the study team's interviewing and facilitating/moderating skills.

The initial training should include guidance on the analysis, interpretation, and documentation of the information gathered. This can be introduced by getting trainees to discuss Chapter 7 of this handbook in particular and linking up the relevant issues raised in Chapters 2 and 4. However, much of the art of carrying out analysis of qualitative data is learned by doing, through on-the-job training during the conduct of investigation.

Management, Review, and Analysis of Information

Qualitative information is analyzed as you collect it. Training should enable the study team to prepare for this time-consuming task. Try reviewing and filing your notes from the training exercises in order to get into the habit of managing data properly. Once the study begins, you will need to review the day's work at the end of each day. Write down ideas as they arise. You will need to organize your notes and put in place a good system for filing information. Advance preparation will help the study to be conducted smoothly. You do not need a computer, although computers can speed up the process of information management and review. Computers can also be hazardous as information can be lost due to power cuts, breakage, and other common mishaps that can happen in the field. In any event, encourage the study team to keep their handwritten notes in folders and notebooks. These can be stored in different ways, and retrieved easily, if a filing system has been carefully prepared.

■ *Keeping notes, notebooks, and files.* Keeping good notes is very important, and these should not only be about things directly related to hygiene practices. Sometimes you do not know what is relevant, so you need to keep comprehensive notes of other things that you feel may be significant. It is also important from the outset of your investigation to identify new questions of relevance to your study, whenever they emerge.

■ *Codes and themes.* Once you have written up detailed notes, mark them up to identify themes that emerge. These can be written as margin notes on the text. For example, you might use CHLDSTO to mark information about the disposal of children's stools, WATSO for water sources, DIARC for causes of diarrhoeal diseases, ACTM for mother's activities, and so on. You need to make up code words that make sense to you, so that when you see a code word, you know immediately whether the text is valuable. But you also need to keep a code book to remind you what the code words stand for. Once the study begins, and by the end of four or five weeks, you may have a lot of codes and may not remember what many of them mean, unless you keep a list of codes at the outset.

You might find a small index book, divided by alphabetical order, especially useful. Organise the code book like a dictionary, and use it only to keep a list of the codes or labels you use for your field notes, interview texts, group discussion transcriptions, and notes. You will need this to check later what certain code terms mean. Avoid complex codes that you might forget, and that others may not be able to decipher.

Developing Working Hypotheses

Many qualitative studies begin by formulating one or more assumptions about possible answers or solutions to the problem(s) to be addressed. In qualitative research these assumptions are called *working hypotheses*, suppositions based on some known facts that serve as starting points for further investigation. Box 6 provides an example of a working hypothesis used in one of the hygiene evaluation studies carried out during the devel-

---

BOX 6
An Example of a Working Hypothesis

In a study conducted in Luoland, Kenya, initial observations of the study villages revealed very little or no faecal contamination in public places: along roads and footpaths or in and around homestead courtyards. At the same time, informal conversations and observations indicated that very few pit latrines in the village were functioning or in use. This led the study team to make the assumption (to hypothesize that):

"There is little or no evidence of faecal contamination in the domestic and public environment despite the absence or lack of use of pit latrines. The reason for this may be that 'digging and burying' is being practiced by everyone."

opment of this handbook. In this particular case, the results of the investigation confirmed the working hypothesis, but this is not a general rule.

Outlining the Study Design

The following are questions to be addressed by the study team as the trainer steers their thinking into designing the planned study.

What is the purpose of the study?
The answer to this question may be:

■ To obtain baseline information on existing hygiene practices prior to intervention.

■ To monitor the progress of hygiene-related interventions by assessing hygiene practices at this point in time.

■ To assess the effectiveness of hygiene-related interventions in changing hygiene practices that had prevailed prior to intervention.

Other purposes may be added depending on the requirements of particular projects.

What types of information will be gathered?
The answer should include some detail on whether the different types of information to be gathered will be qualitative, quantitative, or a combination of both (see Chapter 2).

What is the focus of the study?
Answers to this question will help you develop statements about the *Aims* and *Objectives* of your study (see Chapter 4).

What methods and tools are appropriate?
The following general questions may be asked before choosing suitable methods/tools:

■ Can we learn enough about the practice by asking individual people about it (Interviews)? Will the reported information be sufficient, or

■ Can we learn more about the practice by looking for signs of the behaviour (Observations)? Will it be necessary to choose or develop an *indicator* to *indicate* that the practice has occurred?

■ Can we find out the determinants of these practices by discussions in groups about them (Group Discussions)?

What are the units of analysis?

The units of analysis used and the sampling strategies applied will depend on the type of information gathered in terms of the qualitative-quantitative mix. Whether or not the study is designed to also include quantitative data will depend on the resources available. The need to define units of study or analysis such as community, household, family, has been discussed in Chapter 2. The unit of analysis you choose must reflect your decision as to which group you want to say something about. Are you interested in findings about individuals, groups, or subgroups, such as young children and their caretakers?

Which sampling strategies will be employed?

Are you and the decision makers and other users of the information generated by your study interested in what your study will show about variations among individuals or families or groups? The answer will determine the sampling strategy or strategies you adopt. There are two broad types of sampling strategies: purposeful sampling or probability sampling. In qualitative studies, purposeful sampling is more appropriate than probability sampling, but these are not mutually exclusive categories and some elements of one type of sampling may be found in the other (see "Sampling Strategies" in Chapter 4 for a detailed guide).

How will confidence in the findings be established?

It is crucial to address this question during the processes of designing and planning the study. To be effective, data quality checks need to be put in place early in the design of qualitative investigations (see "Putting in Place Data Quality Checks" in Chapter 4 for a detailed discussion of some of such checks).

When will the study be conducted? How will it be phased?

Will your study involve long-term fieldwork? How will that be phased to fit in with your other project activities? Will the study be designed as a rapid assessment exercise? Is it going to be exploratory with a fixed time frame or an open end? Time issues are discussed further in Chapter 4.

How will logistics be organized?

Practical details related to the logistics of conducting the study are important components of planning and may influence the design of the study. For example, easy access to people and records and availability of training facilities may determine the scope of your study.

How will ethical issues and matters of confidentiality be handled?
In Chapter 2, we discussed issues of ethical relevance. These will also need to be addressed as part of the study design and planning processes.

What resources will be available? What will the study cost?
See Chapter 2 and "Developing Working Hypotheses" in this chapter for guidelines on what to budget for.

Have members of the study team been allocated specific tasks?
By the end of the planning and initial training period, individual members of the study team can be allocated specific tasks, according to their demonstrated skills and/or previous responsibilities. Very often, it is found that one person may excel in doing two or more different things during the training session while another person may seem to be good at only one task. However, the same people may turn out to be the opposite when it comes to carrying out the study. Therefore, task allocations need to be tentative during planning and they should be reviewed when the study begins. Reviewing the capacity of the study team both at the beginning of the study and at regular intervals thereafter will help to identify areas where change of roles/tasks may be required.

What Resources Are Needed?

The resources required for the initial and also for the continuing (on-the-job) training may include the following:

- Resource person(s) with experience in social science research and who are familiar with water supply, sanitation, and hygiene/health education interventions.

- Designated funds to pay for the trainer(s) fees or participants' accommodation and subsistence costs, stationery and photocopying, transportation to the training site and for field visits, refreshments for group discussions, and so on.

- This handbook and other relevant teaching materials (such as those listed in *Selected Reading*) according to the specific needs of the study team.

- Administrative support staff to help with communications (including phone and fax where applicable), photocopying, and so on.

- Stationery (including flip charts, marker pens, notebooks, pens, pencils, glue, adhesive tape, etc.).

- Computers, if available and if required, for information management and documentation/report writing.

- Designated space for training—a school classroom or project office meeting/seminar room. A special venue is helpful: it is not a good idea to train people in their workplaces, where interruptions are possible.

- If there are field trips, then you may have to pay for the use of a vehicle and/or petrol and/or the driver's salary.

- Video films or other visual materials on the use of different methods/tools such as those from PRA, or showing a focus group discussion in session if available; cassette recorders for interviews and/or focus group discussions to allow trainees to practice recording and listening to recorded conversations.

How Much Time Should Be Allowed for Training?

Training of the study team is a continuous process that begins when the team is first formed until the end of the proposed study. This can take anywhere from a few weeks (six to eight weeks) to a few months (three months). For the purposes of the application of this handbook, we have divided the training into two parts: initial training which begins at the preplanning stage, and on-the-job training which continues throughout the conduct of the study. Each project may allow varying lengths of time for each part of the training depending on the availability of time and other resources.

See Table 1 for an example from rural Tanzania where a hygiene evaluation study was conducted. The study team consisted of selected personnel from the three government ministries: Water (*Maji*), Health (*Afya*) and Social Development (*Maendeleo*) assisted by a (WaterAid) resident engineer and a medical anthropologist from outside who conducted the training and study coordination. The intersectoral and interdisciplinary study team was not specially formed for the study. Instead, it was a pre-existing team that had had considerable experience of fieldwork as part of the health education activities supported by WaterAid in Dodoma Region. There were four such teams in the region, one for each district, and two teams were involved in the study which covered two districts.

Training of the WaterAid, *Maji*, *Maendeleo* and *Afya* (WAMMA) teams who participated in the study was done in two phases. The first

TABLE 1

An Example of a Study Timetable Including an Activity Flow Chart

Part I: Preplanning and Initial Training

Days 1–12

- Meetings with project staff

- Discussion of expectations

- Discussion of study aims, objectives and expected outputs

- Visits to the selected study sites—acquisition of consent from concerned parties, including village leaders

- Commencement of initial training

- Discussion of study schedule and preparations for fieldwork

Part II(a): Fieldwork (District I)

Days 1–2 (Project office)

- Resumption of training

- Study design—include choice of methods/tools

Days 3–5 (Village 1)

- Conduct of three-pile sorting, healthwalk, community mapping, historyline and seasonal calendar for illnesses

- On-site review of information

Days 6–7 (Project office)

- Interim review and write up of findings

Days 8–10 (Village 1)

- Feedback to participants—results of historyline and mapping

- Semi-structured interviews, seasonal calendars for activities (gender-specific) and pocket chart

- Feedback to participants—results of seasonal calendar for illnesses and activities, three-pile sorting and pocket chart

Days 11–12 (Project office)

- Interview and observation notes write-up

- Overall review, summary, and discussions

- Discussion of follow-up plans

Part II(b): Fieldwork (District II)

Days 15–16 (Project office)

- Resumption of initial training

- Study design—include choice of methods

Days 17–19 (Village 2)

- Three-pile sorting, historyline, healthwalk, mapping, semi-structured interviews, seasonal calendars, and focus group discussion

- On-site review of information

Days 20–21 (Project office)

- Interim review and documentation of findings

Days 22–23 (Village 2)

- Semi-structured interviews (cont.), three-pile sorting and focus group discussion

- Feedback to participants

- Slide show at village primary school

- Presentation of results to participants

Day 24 (Project office)

- Overall review, write-up of interview and observation notes

- Discussion of preliminary findings and follow-up plans

Day 25 (Project office)

- Joint meeting of two study teams, discussion of study findings and follow-up plans

- End of fieldwork celebration

phase, initial training, involved discussions of the rationale for assessing hygiene practices. Documented references were used to inform the study teams about current research findings and reviews of relevant works in the areas of hygiene behaviour and control of diarrhoeal diseases. The *F diagram* (see Figure 1, Chapter 1) was used in the discussion of sanitation-related disease transmission.

This was followed by a review of the investigative and analytical methods/tools available. The methods and tools with which the WAMMA were already familiar were reviewed before any new ones were introduced. Each WAMMA team reviewed the five clusters of hygiene practices with a view to identifying those that are most relevant for their respective study communities (see Table 2, Chapter 4). The most appropriate methods and tools for assessing the relevant hygiene practices were then selected, discussed, and tried out before the team set out for the study villages.

The initial training also included a detailed discussion of a four-stage learning process: problem identification/defining the question(s), gathering information, reviewing the information, and reflecting on the results. The hygiene evaluation cycle (see Figure 2, Chapter 4) was discussed and frequently referred to throughout the study. The initial training also included trial runs of the selected methods and tools, facilitated by introducing games and role plays including those described in "Transferring Technical Know-How" in this chapter.

The total duration of initial training in this case was two weeks, a week for each team which was located in a different district considerably distant from the other. This is an example of how logistical problems can limit the amount of time allowed for initial training. However, this was not a serious problem in this case because the WAMMA teams both consisted of highly skilled individuals (including district medical officers, community development specialists and public health engineers/technicians) who had already attended related training courses together and were used to working as a team. A week's focused training for each team was thus considered sufficient.

4

Designing a Hygiene Evaluation Study

- *Hygiene Evaluation Cycle*
- *Defining the Objectives of the Study*
- *Developing Specific Objectives*
- *Sampling Strategies*
- *Putting in Place Data Quality Checks*
- *Scheduling Activities*

Hygiene Evaluation Cycle

When developing this handbook, we tried to resolve what we might call the *applied anthropologist's dilemma*. On the one hand, we encourage project staff with little or no previous training in anthropology or related disciplines to be involved in conducting qualitative investigations. This requires practical training and conscientious supervision of project staff. On the other hand, the constraints of time and other resources which project staff face impose limitations on how satisfactorily they can engage in such systematic investigations. Very often, qualitative investigations raise issues that cannot be fully addressed in a short period of time. Can anthropological and related studies be carried out rapidly by study teams with less training than might have been desirable? The answer is yes and no at the same time: the less time available for systematic qualitative investigations, the more highly trained and knowledgeable of the study site and populations the investigators need to be.

The hygiene evaluation studies proposed by the guidelines in this handbook may be carried out rapidly in a matter of a few months, if not weeks. Rapid assessments, however focused, may leave a number of questions unanswered and point to areas where more investigation is required. For this reason, one hygiene evaluation study should not be seen as an end in itself. In a project setting, it may be helpful to visualize one hygiene evaluation study as a cycle within the larger project cycle of planning, monitoring, and measuring impact. It may be necessary to repeat a hygiene evaluation cycle (one study) periodically. The purpose of the repeat studies may be for *follow-up* or further investigation of issues raised by the previous one (for example, issues related to seasonal variation which cannot be addressed by a single study), or for monitoring or measuring impact. This is illustrated by linking up a series of investigations, experiential learning cycles as shown in Figure 2.

Each hygiene evaluation study (one cycle), can be seen as a four-stage learning process:

■ Problem identification/defining the question(s).

■ Gathering information systematically.

■ Reviewing the information.

■ Reflecting on the results and/or taking remedial action.

This was adapted from the principles of experiential learning, or learning by doing (Kolb, 1984). Any one of the above four points may be a starting point for the cycle, although we start with the first one. This cycle represents the different stages of a hygiene evaluation study. [The study team may also find it useful to use the same principles in their daily routine sessions of information gathering, review, interpretation of results, identification of questions for further investigation and information gathering, etc. throughout the study period.]

If the purpose of your study is to measure the impact of project intervention, it may be necessary to add a quantitative component to your study in addition to the qualitative investigation. In that case, you may consider the use of a questionnaire that has been formulated to reflect the findings of your qualitative investigation.

At the end of your study, you will have defined a number of issues to be tackled in the next rapid assessment cycle, that will help complete the picture obtained by the present study. If you are able to follow the cycles of investigation/evaluation, implementation and further investigation in

FIGURE 2
Hygiene Evaluation Cycle
Adapted from Kolb's Experimental Learning Theory (1984)

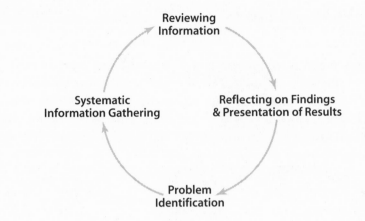

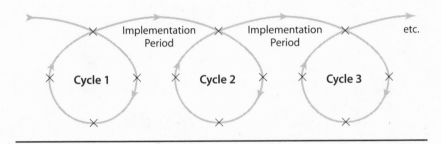

your project work, you will have resolved the problems of incomplete results and limited resources, benefitting from a core study team trained in a piecemeal approach to systematic qualitative investigations.

Defining the Objectives of the Study
The objectives of your study will first depend on its purpose. If, for example, you want to assess the effectiveness of an intervention you have carried out to change particular hygiene practices, then your objectives will include the measurement of change in these specific practices. If, however, you intend to obtain baseline information on existing hygiene practices prior to developing a successful hygiene education intervention, you may want to study a greater range of hygiene practices in order to

find out which are most in need of intervention. The *overall objectives* should be decided in consultation with the expected users of the information gathered in the study—for example, the project managers—and as much as possible with representatives of the study population(s) as well. Study aims and general objectives are closely linked to the study's intended outputs. Box 7 provides an example in which these were defined during the preplanning and initial training phase of a hygiene evaluation study conducted in Kerala, India.

When defining study objectives, you need to consider which *cluster* or *clusters* of hygiene practices to investigate (see Table 2). The number of clusters to consider will be influenced by the purpose of your study and available time and other resources. If time is limited, it may be best to

---

B O X   7

Defining Study Aims, Objectives, and Intended Outputs (an Example)

Kerala Hygiene Evaluation Study

Aims

The primary aim is to assist field personnel of the socioeconomic units (SEU) to design and conduct a hygiene evaluation study in their project areas. The secondary aim is to assess the utility and practicality of the HEP Handbook for the study team.

General Objectives

1. To understand existing water and sanitation related hygiene practices (Clusters A, B, and C) in their cultural, social, economic and physical contexts.

2. To provide the study team with training and first hand experience of a systematic assessment of hygiene practices.

3. To acquaint the study team with the methodology of pretesting a field handbook (the HEP).

4. To define relevant issues for follow-up action and/or further investigation.

Intended Outputs

1. Feedback to the study participants (community members).

2. A core study team with practical skills for assessing hygiene practices systematically.

3. A complete study report for use by the SEUs. This should include a set of practical recommendations and a follow-up action plan.

4. Contributions of examples/case-studies for the Environmental Health Group (EHG) to include in the revised HEP handbook.

5. Simple tools for monitoring the most critical hygiene practices for SEUs to use periodically.

6. Various articles for disseminating the findings to multi-users, e.g., local, regional and national government and non-government institutions, local and global network newsletters such as the SEU newsletters in English and Malayalam, GARNET Hygiene Behaviour Newlsetter, and various practical journals such as the *Natural Resources Forum, Waterlines*, etc.

prioritize and select one or two clusters rather than risk the quality of your study by trying to address too many clusters in a short period of time. For example, in a project where improved water supplies and sanitation are being introduced, it may be preferable to focus on excreta disposal (Cluster A) and water uses (Cluster B), including water sources (Cluster B) if time allows. Such choices need to take into account local conditions, particularly by considering where changes could be most

TABLE 2
A Guide to the Five Clusters of Hygiene Practices

Cluster of Hygiene Practices	Relevant Features and Activities
Sanitation Excreta Disposal (Cluster A)	■ Location of defecation sites ■ Latrine maintenance (structure and cleanliness) ■ Disposal of children's faeces ■ Hand-washing at *critical* times (after cleaning children's bottoms; after handling children's faeces; after defecation ■ Use of cleansing materials
Water Water Sources (Cluster B)	■ Protection of water source(s) ■ Siting of latrines in relation to water source(s) ■ Maintenance of water source(s) ■ Water use at the source(s) ■ Other activities at water source(s) ■ Water collection methods and utensils ■ Water treatment at the source ■ Methods of transporting water
Water Water Uses (Cluster C)	■ Water handling in the home ■ Water storage and treatment in the home ■ Water use (and reuse) in the home ■ Hand-washing at *critical* times (before or after certain activities, including religious rituals) ■ Washing children's faces ■ Bathing (children and adults) ■ Washing clothes
Food Food Hygiene (Cluster D)	■ Food handling/preparation ■ Utensils used for cooking, serving food, feeding young children, and for storing leftover food ■ Hand-washing at *critical* times (before handling food, eating, feeding young children) ■ Reheating of stored food before serving ■ Washing utensils and use of a dish rack
Environment Domestic and Environmental Hygiene (Cluster E)	■ Sweeping of floors and courtyards ■ Household refuse disposal ■ Cleanliness of footpaths, play areas and roads ■ Management of domestic animals (cattle, dogs, pigs, chicken) ■ Drainage of surrounding areas (location of stagnant water and other mosquito breeding sites) ■ Condition of housing

influential in improving the health of the population. It is important to look to the future as well as the present, and link the results to follow-up action that is indicated for the project itself, where changes may need to be made. Plans for future investigations should also be considered (see "Hygiene Evaluation Cycle" in Chapter 4).

Developing Specific Objectives

A choice must be made about which specific hygiene practices will be investigated within each cluster (see Table 2). Within excreta disposal, for example, latrine maintenance and cleanliness, disposal of children's faeces, and hand-washing after defecation could be selected as practices most influential in the prevention of disease. Such choices need to be made with some knowledge and understanding of the local hygiene situation (see Box 8 for an example of specific objectives developed for one of the overall objectives described in Box 7). Note that the selection of specific hygiene practices made while preplanning and designing the study will be provisional, as you may need to modify or change your list

---

BOX 8
Development of Specific Objectives

General Objective

To understand existing water and sanitation-related hygiene practices in their cultural, social, economic, and physical context.

Specific Objectives

Water
1. To locate all existing water sources.

2. To assess existing hygienic condition of water sources.

3. To find out the water collection, storage and handling practices at the source, in transit, and in the home.

4. To find out the reasons for adopting or not adopting certain hygiene practices.

Sanitation
1. To identify existing sanitary facilities

2. To identify existing domestic hygienic practices in the areas of:

    (a) disposal of children's stools;

    (b) hand-washing at *critical* times.

3. To assess the functionality, use, and upkeep of latrines.

once investigation starts and you discover important practices which had not been identified previously.

Your choice of hygiene practices should be influenced by which water/ sanitation-related infections prevail in your study site and which specific practices may be associated with the transmission of these infections. For example, the World Health Organization Control of Diarrhoeal Diseases Programme suggests that it is important to focus on three sets of hygiene practices, rather than include all possible transmission routes. These are:

- safe disposal of human excreta, particularly the faeces of young children and babies, and of people with diarrhoea;

- hand-washing, after defecation, after handling babies' faeces, before feeding and eating, and before preparing food;

- protecting drinking water from faecal contamination, in the home and at the source (WHO, 1993a:8).

It may be possible to investigate the particular practice of interest, for example, water collection and handling practices at the source, by observation. An observer may go to the source and observe people's activities without attracting too much attention. Other hygiene practices and behaviours are harder to observe, for example, adult defecation, as this is a private matter. In such cases, we suggest that indicators or *signs* of behaviour be observed. A number of indicators that are both effective in indicating the occurrence of a particular practice, and relatively easy to assess have been used. These include:

- *Cleanliness, safety, and soundness of latrine structure.* Indicators of use of latrine. People are unlikely to use one that smells, has a shaky and/ or dirty floor, a leaky roof, or is surrounded by bushes where snakes like to nest.

- *Location of latrine in relation to living quarters.* Indicator of use of latrine. One that is situated too close to or too far from the living quarters, or on the wrong side of the courtyard, or on publicly owned land, may not be used much or may not be maintained well for reasons that will be worth investigating.

- *Means of disposal of children's faeces.* Absence of children's faeces in and around the home and/or presence of potties or clean latrines in households indicates the isolation of faecal contamination in and around the home. This can be investigated relatively easily because attention is drawn to children's rather than adults' hygiene practices, to minimize embarrassment.

■ *Turbidity and smell of water at the source and in the home.* Indicator of contamination of water source and lack of protection. Water that looks muddy or unclear at the source and water that smells of rotting leaves or other organic matter may provide clues of contamination. However, it is necessary to observe how it is used (for example, whether it is filtered, or clarified by adding ash or other materials, or boiled or used for non-drinking purposes) and to ask questions about what is observed.

■ *Presence of soap/hand-washing facilities near latrine.* Indicator of hand-washing after defecation.

Sampling Strategies

Sampling is as important to information gathering as it is to the analysis and interpretation of findings. As Miles and Huberman (1994:27) put it, "as much as you might want to, you cannot study everyone everywhere doing everything. Your choices (whom to look at or talk with, where, when, about what, and why) all place limits on the conclusions you can draw, and how confident you and others feel about them." Sampling-related questions that are frequently asked when designing a hygiene evaluation study include:

■ How many people should I include in my study?

■ What criteria should I use for recruiting participants to the study?

■ How many interviews, observations, and group discussions will I need to conduct?

The short answers to these are:

■ As many as can provide adequate answers to your questions.

■ Criteria which reflect the objectives of your study.

■ As many as can provide the information you are looking for, within the limit of resources (human, material, and time) available to you.

Sampling is perhaps the clearest dividing line between quantitative and qualitative investigations. In particular, two sampling-related differences are noteworthy:

■ Qualitative investigations employ *small* sample sizes where a relatively small number of people set in their context are studied indepth. This is unlike quantitative investigations where large numbers of context-free cases are studied in search of statistical significance.

■ Qualitative samples tend to be, in the main, *purposeful* and not *random*. This is partly because the initial definition of the *whole* is more specific, and partly because social processes have a logic and coherence that random sampling would miss out completely.

In quantitative surveys, standardized scales are used so that individuals and groups can be described as showing more or less of some characteristic, for example, knowledge. Everyone is rated on a limited set of predetermined dimensions. Statistical analyses of these dimensions emphasize central tendencies—averages and deviations from those averages. By comparison, qualitative investigations pay particular attention to uniqueness, be it of the individual, the household, or any other unit of analysis. For this reason, the scales used are not standardized. Instead, they are adapted to take individual variations into account, while being sensitive to similarities among people and generalizations about them.

Sampling strategies may appear complicated at first sight. However, this need not be the case if you allow some time for careful planning and detailed consideration of what it is you would like to say something about in your study. As Feuerstein put it simply (1986:69), "sampling means looking closely at part of something in order to learn more about the whole thing." If, for example, you want to find out what the food in a cooking pot tastes like, you can take a spoonful and taste it. You do not have to eat all the food. This type of sampling is fine if there is only one pot of food to taste. However, when discussing sampling from our study population, we need to think in terms of several pots of food which make up a meal. Each pot has to be sampled to find out what the various parts of the meal are. You can then say something about the food in each pot, as well as the meal as a whole. There are different types of sampling that can be applied when studying a population or a community that is made up of diverse component parts, such as ethnic groups, age groups, etc. which may further be differentiated by gender, socioeconomic status, etc.

It is important to distinguish between purposeful and random sampling strategies (see Box 9). The two types of sampling serve different purposes. Often, combined or mixed sampling strategies are employed within the same study in order to answer different questions. For example, purposeful samples are often not prespecified at the beginning of the study. They can evolve during the study. Initial choice of informants/ study participants may lead the investigator to similar and different infor-

BOX 9

Sampling Strategies (Adapted from Patton, 1990)

Type	Purpose
A. Random Probability Sampling	Representativeness: Sample size a function of population size and desired confidence level.
1. Simple Random Sampling	Permits generalization from sample to the population it represents.
2. Stratified Random and Cluster Samplings	Increase confidence in generalizations to particular subgroups or areas.
B. Purposeful Sampling (examples)	Accounting for variability: sample sizes aim for depth rather than breadth of information.
1. Homogeneous Sampling	Focuses, reduces, simplifies variation (e.g., getting eight out of, say, thirty-four mothers aged between twenty and twenty-five yrs to participate in a focus group discussion in their village. Note that this does not mean that their views will not vary, on the contrary).
2. Chain (sequential) Sampling	Identifies cases of interest from people who know people who know which cases are information-rich (e.g., one traditional birth attendant identified as a key-informant may reveal that she knows others like her in the same locality. This may lead to a sequence of additional informants joining the study).
3. Extreme Case Sampling	Learning from unusual manifestations of the phenomenon of interest (e.g., one or two households in a generally contaminated area may be recruited in the study because they display unusually *good* hygiene practices).
4. Typical Case Sampling	Highlights what is normal or average.
5. Random Purposeful Sampling	Adds credibility to sample when potential purpose is too wide.
6. Stratified Purposeful Sampling	Illustrates subgroups; facilitates comparisons.
7. Criterion Sampling	All cases that meet some criterion; useful for qualitative measurement (e.g., mothers/caretakers of children under five years of age fulfil the criteria of engaging in several hygiene practices as part of their daily routine work).

mants; observing one cluster of hygiene practices may invite comparison with another cluster; and understanding one key relationship in one setting may reveal issues to be addressed in other settings.

More than one sampling strategy can be applied in two different ways: working from the outside into the core of a setting, or working from the core into the wider context of the issue at hand. For example, in studying hygiene practices, you may begin with the study population (use census data, walk around the settlement areas) and then enter the selected villages or sections of towns and the households, staying several days to get a sense of the frequency and occurrence of different events. From there, the focus would be on specific events, times and locations. Alternatively, you may observe a specific practice in one locality and work towards investigating the wider context by looking at neighbouring and more distant localities (see Miles and Huberman, 1994 and Patton, 1986 for more examples and detailed discussions of qualitative sampling issues).

In summary, there are two important steps you need to follow when deciding how many people to include in your study and what criteria you should use for including them:

Step 1: Define the population boundaries of your study site. You may have existing boundaries to distinguish areas where your project activities are currently going on from those that have not had any intervention yet, or those where your project work has already finished. Alternatively, you may find it more useful to define your study population according to political/administrative boundaries such as region, district, division, location or sub-location; according to income levels such as high, middle, and low-income.

Step 2: Find out how many different parts or groups make up the whole, and determine their relevance to the questions your study is aiming to address. You can then take samples or representations of the whole to include in your study.

The example in Box 10 illustrates how samples were recruited according to the purpose of the study, the type of questions addressed, and the indicators used in a hygiene evaluation study. In this case, the working hypothesis was that faecal contamination in and around the home and the hygiene practices associated with them are more prevalent and therefore easier to observe in homesteads with young children than in those without. Participants to group discussions were invited and grouped purposefully.

Putting in Place Data Quality Checks

Processes of checking the quality or trustworthiness of information obtained by using qualitative methods differ from those applied to data obtained from quantitative surveys. *Trustworthiness* checks for qualitative

BOX 10

Some Examples of Purposeful Sampling

The purpose of a trial hygiene evaluation study conducted in Tanzania was to carry out an exploratory assessment of hygiene practices among two selected rural populations. Observations conducted before the study began showed that there were more hygiene-related activities in households with young children than in those without, so only such households were selected for further observation. Informal interviews with the mothers/caretakers of infants and young children were conducted in the same households. The number of interviews and observations in each site was twenty. This number was decided on the basis of the following considerations:

■ Estimated number of households with young children.

■ Total time allocated for interviews and observations in relation to group discussions conducted with participatory visual aids.

The participants of group discussion sessions were self-selected, that is, the groups consisted of those who were willing and able to attend meetings called by the study team. Special efforts were made by the team to invite different categories of people to attend group discussion meetings by visiting homes and explaining the purpose of the meetings to as many people as possible. Participants of group discussions were sometimes divided into sub-groups according to gender, age, and social status.

information are essentially components of study design and execution which enhance the quality or *goodness* of the information gathered. They are not a set of tests to be applied to the data once collected (unlike statistical significance or *goodness-of-fit* tests), but in-built checks that are put in place before the start of data collection and monitored throughout the conduct of investigation. Such checks include:

■ *Prolonged or intense engagement of the various participants.* If you have ample time and other resources required for an extended study, you can check the quality of information you gather through prolonged engagement with the different stakeholders. If, however, the time allowed for a hygiene evaluation study is limited to a few weeks or months, as is often the case in water supply, sanitation and health/ hygiene education projects, you will opt for intensive interaction with the study participants. This requires you to build trust and rapport with the study population, to learn the particulars of the context relatively quickly, and to be open to multiple influences. Trust and rapport can only be established quickly if you already know the local language, understand the cultural nuances and have genuine respect for local people and their ways of life (see "Sensitizing the Study Team" in Chapter 3 for more detail on building rapport).

If your hygiene evaluation study is one of a series of intensive engagements with the study population, that is, one hygiene evaluation cycle to be followed by another (see "Hygiene Evaluation Cycle" in Chapter 4), then you may have both intense and prolonged engagement which will increase the trustworthiness of your findings.

■ *Triangulation of sources, methods, and investigators.* Crosschecking of information on the same topic gathered from different sources, using different methods and/or by different investigators, is an integral part of qualitative investigation. The term *triangulation* derives from land surveying, where bearings are taken by drawing lines from at least two landmarks, in different directions, and finding their intersection point (Patton, 1990:187–9). A given problem can be thoroughly investigated only if information is collected from more than one source, when more than one method or tool of investigation is used, and/or when more than one investigator (with different perspectives) is involved. You can put in place means for triangulation of information by including people with different perspectives in your study team and by combining different methods/tools of investigation (see Table 3 at the end of Chapter 5, and Table 4 at the end of Chapter 6).

■ *Parallel investigations and team communications.* If your study covers more than one location, and you have more than one study team, the teams can crosscheck the quality of each other's data sets by meeting regularly. If all teams are using the same methods, this will enable you to check how replicable the methods are. For parallel investigations to succeed, good communication between team members is important. This requires regular formal meetings and established group norms of behaviour.

■ *Diary of activities.* Each member of the study team should keep a diary of activities throughout the period of preplanning, training, study design, and execution. These may or may not be revealed to others, but will help you at a later stage to remember the immediate reasons for methodological decisions and changes of direction.

■ *Participant checking.* Periodic feedback sessions will enable you to present results of the investigation to members of the study population, and to test whether they agree with your understanding of what they are doing. This will enhance your rapport with them as it demonstrates your interest in their views and comments on your findings.

It will also set in motion ideas for the study participants to implement your findings.

■ *Report(s) with working hypothesis(es), contextual descriptions and visualizations.* Study reports which include sufficiently detailed or *thick* descriptions with visual materials and direct quotations capturing personal perspectives and experiences provide infinitely better checks of data quality than *thin* reports which present information that may be only partially set in context.

■ *Peer review/checking.* Peer reviews allow colleagues (not directly involved in your study) to explore important aspects of the study that might have been overlooked by the team of investigators. This will also help to keep members of the study team honest, by exposing them to searching questions which probe biases and explore meanings.

■ *Impact on stakeholder's capacity to know and act.* As a result of the study processes and outcomes, the study team and other stakeholders should have an increased awareness and appreciation of the issues addressed by the study. This should enable them to plan and execute follow-up action. If those who were involved in the study from the beginning remain unaffected or no wiser about the implications of the results at the end, then you have failed. The level of awareness and appreciation of the study results by those who participated in it ultimately depends on the level of their participation, not only in information gathering but also in the analysis, interpretation, reflection and judgement of the results (see Chapter 7).

Scheduling Activities

In the next chapter, we describe a number of methods and tools you can use for gathering and analysing information. Some of these involve group activities, others are individual observations and interviews to be conducted during home visits. It is useful to plan activities in advance even if you end up having to make some changes when you start gathering information. A good activity plan allows for unforeseen events and includes substitute activities in case of mishap. Some flexibility will be necessary. It is necessary for the planned activity flow-chart to take account of the following considerations:

■ *Ways of maintaining participant's interest and the study team's interest and stamina.* For example, by alternating group activities with individual interview and observations, information gathering with review (with and without participants), and feedback sessions. This can prevent fatigue and lack of motivation/interest while participants and investigators are engaged in intensive interaction. Qualitative investigations demand a lot of energy and stamina. Investigators need to keep alert almost all the time. Make sure you include periodic breaks and days off to allow members of the study team to rest, to refresh their minds, and/or to spend time with their families, especially if they have young children whom they have to leave behind while they travel to the study site(s). Try to correspond these with participant's holidays or busy days such as market days, Fridays or Sundays, and so on.

■ *Available time and resources.* Project personnel often engage in several tasks at the same time, albeit for very short periods of time (a few days at a time), and they may commit themselves to the study, or be asked to do other jobs as well. It is important to think ahead and plan your study carefully to avoid unnecessary interruptions once you start. Interferences can put at risk the study team's motivation and its rapport with the study population(s).

(See Diagram 2. Arrows on the lines and loops indicate interconnections between the various decisions, statements, and activities/processes.)

DIAGRAM 2
Planning Flow Chart

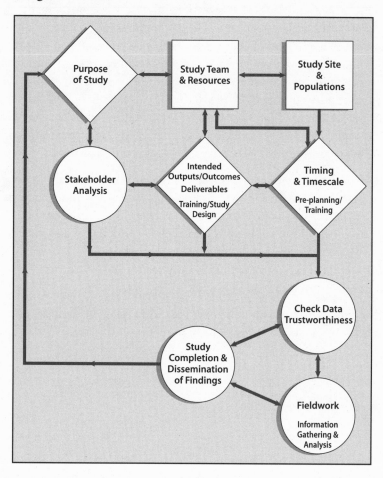

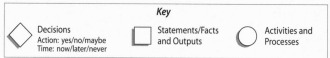

5

Methods and Tools for Investigating the Context

- *Healthwalk (Systematic Walkabout)*
- *Structured (Spot-check) Observations*
- *Key-informant Interviewing*
- *Historyline*
- *Community Mapping*
- *Seasonal Calendar*
- *Gender Roles/Tasks Analysis*
- *Appraisal of the Methods and Tools*

To understand hygiene and sanitation issues fully, it is necessary to explore people's ideas, beliefs and knowledge, and their activities. There are many different ways to collect information on the sociocultural and physical context in which hygiene practices occur. For example, it is not enough to describe existing methods of excreta disposal or people's personal hygiene practices, such as hand-washing, without finding out what physical, social, cultural, or economic constraints might be operating locally to cause people to do what they do. People in the study population can be involved in the investigation, analysis, and interpretation of their own situation. This is important, because they will then have an interest in, and a sense of ownership of the information gathered, and they will perhaps have an interest in making use of the study findings if they are presented in accessible forms.

This chapter describes some of the investigative and analytical tools we have found to be very useful for investigating the context in which hygiene practices occur, and the methods for using those tools. It may be worth noting the distinction made between the terms *method* and *tool*. Method refers to the way of doing something while tool refers to the instrument used for doing it. For example, a questionnaire is an instrument for collecting information and different methods can be applied when using it: it can be used by the respondent to fill in the answers to the questions herself or himself (self-reporting method), it can be administered by an interviewer who asks the questions and marks the answers given by the respondent on a precoded sheet (formal method), or it can be used as a guide by an interviewer who asks open-ended questions for the respondent to answer in an unstructured way (informal method). A description of each tool (including materials used apart from notebooks and pens which each member of the study team should have) and the method of using it (set of procedures) is provided. You will find that some tools, such as observation and interview schedules, are used for information gathering while others such as Maps, seasonal calendars and historylines are created during information gathering and are more participatory. These participatory tools have wider uses:

- They facilitate feedback of the findings to the study population, thereby ensuring participant checking of the information.

- They provide accessible ways of storing/documenting study findings for reference in future investigations or follow-up action.

- They can be used for monitoring project activities and changes in hygiene practices.

There are many more participatory tools that can be used in the investigation and analysis of hygiene practices. This handbook is by no means exhaustive of available methods/tools. The methods/tools described can be adapted and modified to suit particular situations and are thus flexible. What is important is that each method and tool that you use is described carefully and the information obtained is analyzed rigorously. You may also wish to communicate your experiences with these methods/tools or adaptations thereof (see Evaluation Sheet at the end of this handbook). At the end of this Chapter and the next you will find appraisals of each method/tool described (see Tables 3 and 4). This will help you choose and combine methods/tools informedly.

Healthwalk (Systematic Walkabout)

This method is an adaptation of *transect* (a method within Participatory Rural Appraisal, PRA) in which the study team spends one to four hours (depending on distances to be covered) walking across the study site(s) in a meandering fashion. It is essential for the study team, in pairs or triplets (not too many in a group to avoid attracting unnecessary attention), to absorb the atmosphere of the study site as they walk up and down the roads and foot-paths, stopping to greet people of all walks of life. Spontaneous informal conversations and discussions on water and sanitation-related topics may be held, especially where people normally gather: for example, at the water source(s), village/town square, or the market place. This may provide opportunities to identify key-informants, individuals who are particularly knowledgeable about issues relevant to your study, for example, handpump attendants, traditional doctors, birth attendants, water committee chairpersons, and so on (see "Key-Informant Interviewing" below).

Purpose

- To familiarize yourself with the physical context in which hygiene practices occur. This is often done with specific objectives, such as finding out where the water sources are and to assess levels of visible faecal contamination in the public as well as the domestic environment.

- To observe how people behave and interact with each other as they go about their daily routines of fetching water, tilling the land, caring for young children, tending animals, cleaning their homes and courtyards, and so on. This provides some insight into what people do when they are not at meetings, for instance.

Tool

A checklist of what to look out for—a spot-check observation schedule—is often used (see the example in "Structured (Spot-Check) Observations" below).

Procedure

- Conduct the healthwalk at dawn and/or dusk. Most of the relevant hygiene practices occur very early in the mornings or in the late afternoon/early evenings. It is unlikely that you will observe many of the relevant activities in the middle of the day. Conduct healthwalks at both times of day if time allows. Be careful to observe local customs and social rules. For example, in predominantly Islamic communities, such as those in rural Afghanistan, it is not acceptable for women to walk about and talk to people they do not know. Members of the study team may, in such cases, be allocated tasks that are suitable/ acceptable for their gender.

■ Familiarize yourself with the tool before you set out on the healthwalk, and use it discreetly, as a reminder, if you need to refer to it during the healthwalk. Do not wave it around during the heathwalk as it might arouse suspicion among the people you meet.

■ Look, listen, and learn.

■ Jot down details of what you observed, and make notes of things that were said during conversations with people you met (see Box 11).

■ Use this opportunity to meet people who may not normally go to meetings, for example, mothers and/or caretakers of young children. Explain to them the purpose of your visit or stay in the area, and invite them to participate in your meetings.

■ Be careful not to make mistakes that may endanger your rapport with the study population (see Box 12).

BOX 11

An Extract of Notes from a Healthwalk

From the Rift Valley town of Meki, Ethiopia

...The study team proceeded to the public water standpost where the attendant/fee-collector had promised to be by 8:30. A number of women came to fetch water and when they saw that there was no sign of the attendant (a young man) anywhere near the standpost, proceeded to a water vending place on the main road—a shop that had a piped water connection and was selling water at the same price as the public standpost. The study team observed a young man buying water with a big barrel which he was going to transport using a wheel-barrow. The barrel was about 300 litres capacity and he paid sixty cents for it. On returning to the public standpost, the same children who had pushed their wheel barrows with a few jerrican water containers were waiting for the attendant to come and open the public standpost. It was almost 9:00 and there was no sign of him. The study team decided to go and look for him at the WSSA offices...He said that he "had more important things to do at the WSSA office" that morning which was why he was late. When the study team mentioned that they were interested in talking with the water users about the situation of water supply in Meki, he said dismissively, *"Inesu yemiawkut neger ale bilachihu new?"* which roughly translates as, "So you think they know anything about it, do you?" The study team noted his arrogance and uncooperative manner both towards them and towards the water users.

BOX 12

Examples of Common Mistakes Made on a Healthwalk

- A member of the study team opened the door of a latrine in one compound, saw that it was dirty, and turned around immediately, slamming the door behind her. The lady of the house, an expectant mother whose hands were covered in soil as she had just returned from her *shamba* was visibly embarrassed by this reaction. The lady explained that she had only just returned from working in the gardens and that she had not had time to clean the latrine.

- A member of the study team arrived in the compound of a homestead where other members of the team were already engaged in a conversation with homestead owners. Instead of allowing the conversation to continue after greeting them, she immediately started asking her own questions, some of which had already been asked by the other team members.

Information Management and Review

At the end of this exercise, you should meet with your study team to discuss your notes and observations. You will find that the combined notes and observations make for a detailed data set on both general and specific issues. The notes will include information which may be clearly relevant or significant as well as trivial detail. Summarize your data, noting any observations that appear intriguing, revealing or relevant, to the questions you aim to address in your study. You may also want to formulate further questions for investigation. It is good practice to keep all your notes until the end of the study although you may be tempted to throw away field notes which appear to be irrelevant to your objectives. It is possible that when you get to the overall analysis stage, you will find an explanation to an intriguing finding hidden in field notes that had been put aside.

Information collected during a healthwalk can thus be used by the study team to:

- formulate or redefine questions to be addressed in the study in the light of what has been seen and heard;

- identify ways to reach different categories of study participants, such as busy mothers/caretakers of young children, community elders, and leaders, through appropriate communication channels;

- interpret findings at the end of your investigations;

- make decisions on issues related to project design and implementation.

For example, the example cited in Box 11 had an immediate impact on the project concerned (see Box 13 for the project managers' description of how healthwalk data were used).

BOX 13

An Example of Implementation of Information Gathered During a Healthwalk

Supplied by the Manager of the Project Concerned

"Decision criteria adopted by engineers are, all too often, based on figures utilized for previous projects of a similar nature and tend not to be specific for the actual scheme in question. A fundamental principal of the Twelve Towns Water Supply and Sanitation Study carried out by GIBB in Ethiopia was that the solutions proposed for each town should be entirely appropriate for the local population. While underdesign would result in project objectives not being achieved, overdesign could result in an expensive scheme which is unattractive to potential financing agencies and one which would overload the operation and maintenance capabilities of the local authorities. It is essential that water is supplied at the locations and quantities required and that it is available at an acceptable and affordable price. Failure could result in the local population resorting to traditional sources which are generally polluted and distant from the town.

"In order to achieve this target, actual water and sanitation related hygiene practices were evaluated utilizing methods outlined in this handbook, together with an indepth evaluation of the ability of the local population to pay for water utilized. The end result was a project which provided the appropriate amount of water at required locations with a realistic division between the standard supply categories of house connections, yard connections, and public fountains. In the case of the town of Meki, the engineers analysing the existing water supply system picked up on the problems associated with the standpost, and determined via computer simulation of the supply network, that enforcement of proper operator working hours would increase the volume of water available to the public by approximately 30%."

Structured (Spot-Check) Observations

Observation is a standard anthropological method for gathering information. It is a relatively unobtrusive and highly effective method that is often combined with other methods, such as interviewing. Observations can be done in a structured way, using a set of preselected things to observe, or in an unstructured manner by noting down everything observed and then classifying the information according to relevant themes. When the study objectives are specific, clearly defined, and the time allowed for the study is limited, as is often the case in assessments of hygiene practices, structured observations are more appropriate than unstructured ones. Spot-check observations are the simplest type of structured observations that can be conducted during a healthwalk, as well as during household visits and when interviewing.

Purpose

- To see where water and sanitation-related facilities are located and to obtain first hand information on hygiene practices in and around these locations.

■ To find out about hygiene-related practices in and around people's homes.

Tool

A structured (often precoded) spot-check observation schedule may be prepared, that consists of a list of relevant things to look for. This should reflect local features and may be pretested during the training period (see Chapter 3). An example which was adapted for different settings and translated into the local languages during the development and testing of this handbook is included (see Worksheet 1). Make your own guide to suit your particular setting, and do not be confined to this example.

Procedure

■ Study the structured observation schedule well before conducting the observations. Use the skills you learned during the initial training (see Chapter 3).

■ Be mentally prepared—concentrate.

■ Try to be unobtrusive—for example, do not wave your checklist around or draw unnecessary attention to what you are doing.

■ Look, listen, and learn.

■ Write down your observations. All additional information to what is listed on the spot-check observation schedule should be included in your written notes with as much relevant detail as possible.

Management, Review, and Use of Information

Discuss everyone's observation notes in your study team and sort them by general themes and specific clusters of hygiene practices. Prepare a summary and keep it safe for crosschecking against information obtained by other methods in the final/overall analysis and inclusion in your study report. Define questions for further investigation arising from your discussion.

Key-Informant Interviewing

Key-informant interviewing is a standard anthropological method which is widely used in health-related investigations (see Pelto and Pelto, 1978). The term key-informant may be used for anyone who can provide you with detailed information, on the basis of their special expertise or knowledge of a particular issue. For example, a local health worker is the ideal

Worksheet 1

An Example of a Structured Observation Guide Used During a Healthwalk

Water

1. What are the available water sources?
   (a) well
   (b) spring
   (c) reservoir/dam
   (d) rain water
   (e) seasonal pond
   (f) public stand post/tap/fountain
   (g) hand-dug well
   (h) other

2. Are the water sources protected? (indicate which ones)
   (a) yes
   (b) semi-protected
   (c) no

3. How far are water sources from people's homes?

Water source   Distance
_____ (a) less than 100 meters
_____ (b) 100–500 meters
_____ (c) less than 1 km
_____ (d) 1–2 km
_____ (e) 3–5 km
_____ (f) 6–7 km
_____ (g) more than 8 km

4. What activities take place at or near the water source?
   (a) washing water containers
   (b) washing clothes
   (c) bathing/washing self
   (d) watering animals
   (e) other

5. Who collects water?
   (a) women
   (b) children
   (c) men

6. What utensils (and means) are used for fetching water?

7. How is water transported from the source to the home?

8. Is water treated at the source, and if so, how?
   (a) by filtering with a piece of cloth
   (b) by chlorination
   (c) by other means

*9. How is drinking water stored in the home?

*10. How is drinking water handled in the home?

* Can also be used during during household visits, in conjunction with semi-structured interviews.

Sanitation

1. Is there evidence of faecal contamination?
   (a) along the roads?
   (b) along the foot-paths?
   (c) near the water source?
   (d) in/near the fields/*shambas*?
   (e) outside the houses?
   (f) inside the houses?

2. What is the contamination observed?
   (a) infants/young children's faeces
   (b) adults' faeces
   (c) cow dung and/or other animal faeces
   (d) other

3. Did you see anyone defecating? (Who? Where? Describe)

4. How many of the houses you visited have latrines?

*5. Where is the latrine located? (indicate reasons why, if relevant)
   (a) inside the courtyard
   (b) outside the courtyard

*6. Observe the latrine.
   (a) Does it have a sound super-structure?
   (b) Is the floor safe to stand on?
   (c) Does it have a slab?
   (d) Is the hole small enough to be safe for children?
   (e) Does the latrine provide adequate privacy?
   (f) Any other features?

*7. Is the latrine in use?
   (a) Is the path leading to it clear?
   (b) Is it clean?
   (c) Is it reasonably free of smell?
   (d) Are there cleansing materials in the vicinity? What are they?
   (e) Is there water in the vicinity?
   (f) Is there ash in the vicinity?
   (g) Any other evidence of use?

*8. How close are hand-washing facilities (water and ash or soap) to the latrine?
   (a) next to the latrine
   (b) within walking distance
   (c) inside the house

* Can also be used during during household visits, in conjunction with semi-structured interviews.

key-informant to talk to you about infections, but not necessarily about other matters concerning water and sanitation. A village leader or village health volunteer could be helpful when discussing community participation projects. Women may be ideal key informants to discuss children's defecation habits, and so on. Who you choose as a key-informant depends on the topic that interests you at the time. The investigator would simply raise a topic for conversation with the respondent, then let the respondent take the lead. If the respondent is highly knowledgeable on the subject raised, she or he can become a key-informant.

Key-informant interviewing at the beginning of the study may help you to gain a good overview of the relevant issues. You can then begin to develop question lines for focus group discussions, identify issues to cover in observations, and so on. The subject of an interview may be very broad, such as health, or farming, or family structures in the locality; or it may be more specific—which water sources are best for which purposes, for example. Key-informant interviewing can thus provide valuable information on both specific hygiene practices and on the context in which they are assessed.

Management, Review, and Use of Information
The management of key-informant review notes, their review/analysis, and use is the same as that described in "Semi-Structured (Informal) Interviews" in Chapter 6.

Historyline
This method is an adaptation of PRA's *Timeline* which is used for gathering time-related information. This method is good for establishing good relations between the study team and the participants, as it instills confidence in local people, particularly community elders. Often, investigators consult community leaders and forget to involve the elders who may be more knowledgeable about the history of their locality. Historyline involves such knowledgeable people (who may include individuals identified as key-informants) in a group discussion and analysis of local history, thereby reinforcing the value of their knowledge.

Purpose
■ To investigate local history in general terms, e.g., by learning about local, regional, national, and international events that are considered by local people to be important.

■ To investigate specific issues related to the management of natural resources such as water, land, and fuel.

This method is good for building rapport as it instills confidence in local people, particularly community elders, by involving them in a way that makes them see that their knowledge counts.

Materials
Use locally available materials, such as a stick for sketching a straight line on the ground, and stones or leaves for marking events or names of chiefs on the line, the historyline. The dates or names representing memorable events are marked on the historyline.

Procedure
■ Invite local elders to meet with at least two members of the study team for consultation about the history of the area.

■ Explain to the elders that you are interested to learn about important events that have taken place in the past and may or may not have been written down before. Assure them that your intention is to learn and not to judge, and that you are not going to use the information they provide against them.

■ Listen and learn.

■ Encourage every participant to contribute. Ask for further explanation of anything that is not clear to you. Ask for confirmation if you feel unsure whether you have understood what you have been told, or if the information given seems surprising or conflicting.

■ When the historyline chart and discussion are complete, summarize the results verbally and ask the participants if the information you have presented reflects the discussion correctly, and note their responses. Thank everyone for their contribution and bring the meeting to a close. You may wish to serve refreshments, if available.

■ Present the historyline chart to a larger group of study participants at another time. For example, you could start your next group discussion by giving feedback on what you have learned about local history using the historyline. This serves to stimulate participants' interest in the study.

Management, Review, and Use of Information

The historyline should be transferred to paper for the study team to discuss. This may be done using a flip chart where the historyline can be drawn, showing the appropriate dates, names, and other captions. A detailed account of what was said at the meeting may be written down separately. See Figure 3 and Box 14 for an example of a historyline constructed in the Dodoma region, Kondoa district of Tanzania. In this example, a historyline was used to investigate why Kwayondu village, which has chronic water shortages, was chosen by the early settlers and the answer was provided almost as soon as the meeting began. Six village elders participated in constructing the historyline which was later presented and verified at a large meeting.

The historyline chart can be used as a reference as well as a monitoring tool in follow-up activities. For example, local community groups may

---

BOX 14

Extract of Notes Taken During the Discussion of a Historyline

From Kwayondu village, Tanzania

According to the *wazee*, village elders, the place which is now known as Kwayondu village was originally called Yoyo because a long time ago, two men were trying to cross the river in that region and one of them was carried off by the floods and subsequently drowned. Shocked by this event, the surviving man shouted " yoyo!" until people could hear him. One of the elders could remember hearing about this incident and about Yoyo around 1947. It was agreed that 1947 could be the starting point.

In 1948, the colonial government built a cattle trough to prepare the place for settlement. This cattle trough was receiving water from Kandaga spring [through a gravity scheme]. In 1949, most of the people from Chakwe, a village near Kondoa town, were forcibly moved to Kwayondu. The elders explained that this was not a sudden event. It had been premeditated by the colonial government. Some time before the move, the government had prepared the area for settlement by paying some people to clear the forest as part of a tsetse fly control project and built many *tembe* huts, made of wattle and swab with flat roofs. The people of Chakwe were then transported by government trucks to the new place and were told "These will be your huts. You will live here," when they reached Kwayondu. The new village was full of mosquitoes, so much so that the people could not sleep inside their huts at night. They slept on the roofs of the *tembe*. One of the elders recalled that he was a young boy at that time and one night while he was asleep, he fell down from the roof and broke his arm. He showed everyone at the meeting the scar on his arm which had resulted from that fall.

The village was named Kwayondu because it had many Baobab trees with beehives on them. The beehives belonged to a man called Yondu. *Mzee* Yondu lived in Bukulu, a distant village close to the western border of Bereko Division. When he saw that the area where he kept his hives was being cleared, he appealed to the colonial government to spare the Baobab trees. He went to see the District Commissioner (DC), taking with him some of the honey from the Baobab trees. The DC agreed to spare the Baobab trees, and so they stand to this day...

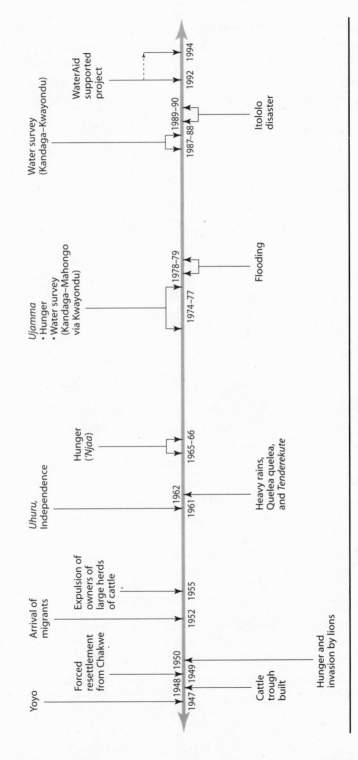

FIGURE 3

Historyline of Kwayondu Village, Tanzania
(Number of Participants/Informants = 6 Elders)

want to keep a copy of it as a record of information that had not been previously documented. It may also serve as a project monitoring tool in a follow-up study. The example in Figure 3 can be used to monitor the progress of the WaterAid-supported water supply project and can be updated at given intervals.

Community Mapping

This method also derives from PRA and is widely used as part of other types of participatory approaches as well. Participants are asked to create a *map*, a representation of their territory, showing places that are important to them (marketplaces, mosques, churches, etc.) and including features of interest to the investigator(s), such as water sources and sanitation facilities.

Purpose

■ To find out what public facilities related to health and hygiene to which the community has access, such as where people draw water from.

■ To find out about hygiene and sanitation resources in people's homes (latrines, rubbish pits, dishracks, etc.). This may include items that have been introduced or promoted by your project.

Materials

These will depend on the resources available. Maps can be made using sticks to sketch on the ground and placing stones and leaves to mark important places. If participants are familiar with using pens and paper and you can afford them, these can be used. Other alternatives are flip charts and marker pens, or blackboard and chalk.

Procedure

The following guidelines may be useful to the facilitator:

■ Introduce yourself and explain the purpose of the meeting and the planned activity. Speak clearly, in the local language.

■ Explain the task. Allow ample time for the participants to discuss the concept of a map, to ask questions, and to make suggestions as to how they would go about drawing it and what materials they want to use. (Sometimes villagers do not want to use sticks and stones, choosing instead pencil and paper, or chalk and blackboard.)

■ Listen, look, and learn.

■ Encourage/stimulate discussion, but do not dictate what should and should not be on the map.

■ Keep a list of participants to refer to later, when checking the information on the map against similar information obtained using other tools.

■ When the map is finished, show it to the whole group and ask people to discuss any changes they think need to be made.

■ Present the map to a larger group of study participants at another time. For example, you could start your next group discussion by giving feedback on what you have learned about local features and hygiene-related facilities using the map. This serves to stimulate participants' interest in the study.

Management, Review, and Use of Information

The map will contain information both about physical features of the locality and about people's attitudes to it. Often the process of making the map and finding out about the local context through the discussions is just as important as the information on the map itself.

Maps can provide information that is easily quantifiable. For example, the number of homesteads in a village and even the hygiene-related facilities in each courtyard can be shown (for example, see Figure 4 which shows map from two villages in western Kenya where a number of facilities for improved hygiene, promoted by the SHEWAS project, were indicated). Information from these maps was tabulated as shown in Box 15. This helped the study team make informed sampling decisions for semi-structured interviews with mothers of young children. Here the number of homesteads in the two villages was found to be the same, but the

---

BOX 15

An Example of Quantifiable Information Obtained from the Maps Shown on Figure 4

Features and Indicators	Haudinga	Masanga
Homesteads (clusters of households)	33	33
Homesteads with young children	20	21
Latrines inside the compound	4	1
Latrines outside the compound	17	25
Washstands (for hand-washing after latrine use)	2	9

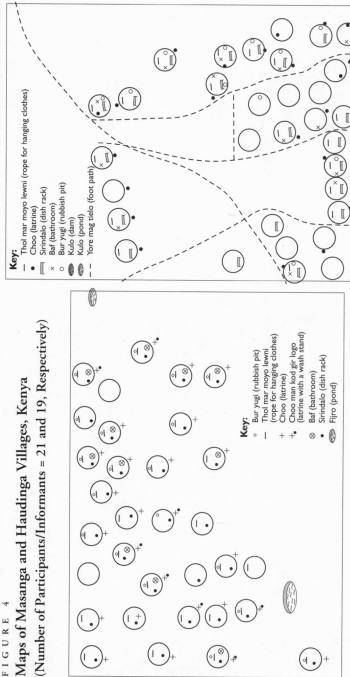

F I G U R E   4
Maps of Masanga and Haudinga Villages, Kenya
(Number of Participants/Informants = 21 and 19, Respectively)

Key:
— Thol mar moyo lewni (rope for hanging clothes)
• Choo (latrine)
▦ Sirindalo (dish rack)
× Baf (bathroom)
○ Bur yugi (rubbish pit)
○ Kulo (dam)
◉ Kulo (pond)
– – Yore mag tielo (foot path)

Key:
○ Bur yugi (rubbish pit)
— Thol mar moyo lewni
   (rope for hanging clothes)
+ Choo (latrine)
⁺• Choo man kod gir logo
   (latrine with a wash stand)
⊗ Baf (bathroom)
• Sirindalo (dish rack)
◉ Fijro (pond)

from Tom Mboya's (SHEWAS Project) copy of the original

number of families or households in each homestead/courtyard ranged from six to ten. However, the most valuable part of mapmaking is often not the tabulated information, but the analysis provided during the discussion of the maps, which helps to interpret the numbers and to understand their significance.

In some cases maps can include politically sensitive detail such as the marking of boundaries (see Box 16).

The map can be used as a monitoring tool for future assessments. As is the case with a historyline, the map can serve as a document in which a record can be kept of what existed at the time of your study. The map should be dated so that when revisiting the area and conducting follow-up assessments of hygiene practices, any changes that have taken place can be noted by comparing maps. For example, a map created two years after the ones shown in Figure 4 might show that several latrines have been constructed inside the homestead courtyards as a result of some solution arrived at by community members to get around the existing cultural taboo prohibiting in-laws from sharing latrines.

Seasonal Calendar

This method also originates from PRA and is used for the purposes of presenting large quantities of diverse information in a common time frame. Using this method, local people's accounts of the seasonal pattern of rainfall, agricultural labour (usually differentiated by gender), illness, etc., can be represented visually using local materials.

Purpose

■ To obtain detailed information on the activities of local men, women, and children at different times of the year.

BOX 16

An Example of Sensitive Issues that Can Arise in Mapmaking

From Kwayondu Village, Tanzania

Some community members were concerned about the village boundaries as they appeared on the map of *Kitongoji A* (a section of the village). They explained [to members of the study team] that they were currently involved in a dispute with the inhabitants of a neighbouring village about ownership of some of the land on the boundary between the two villages. The case had been taken to court and was still unresolved. The map presented by the study team seemed to support their opponent's side. After discussing this problem at length, the participants accepted this map, but urged the study team not to show it to anyone in the neighbouring village as it might be used in evidence against them.

■ To find out which illnesses are perceived to be most important and at what time of year or season they are most prevalent.

A ranking system can be used for the study participants to indicate whether a given activity in a given month is of low, medium, or high intensity. Similarly, climatic indicators such as rainfall and temperature may be graded high, medium, and low, and the prevalence of the most important/common illnesses can be graded in the same way.

Materials
The materials required for this tool are the same as those described for mapping above.

Procedure

■ Introduce yourself and your team and explain to participants the purpose of the meeting.

■ Instructions should be given clearly, in the local language(s), and you should allow ample time for the participants to discuss the local calendar, ask questions, and choose the materials they want to use. Assure participants that you are there to learn, not to judge or give advice.

■ Listen (and look) and learn.

■ Encourage everyone to contribute and allow for each contribution to be discussed.

■ Keep a participants list to enable you to check who they were when reviewing the data.

■ After completion, transfer the chart to a flip chart or black board, present it to the study participants, and invite their comments and suggestions. Any necessary corrections and alterations can be made on-site.

■ Present the seasonal calendar(s) to a larger group of study participants at another time. For example, you could start your next group discussion by giving feedback on what you have learned about local climate, illnesses, and activities using the seasonal calendar(s). This serves to stimulate participants' interest in the study.

Management, Review, and Use of Information
You can store data obtained from a seasonal calendar on bar charts accompanied by the interpretation in text form (see, for example, Figure 5

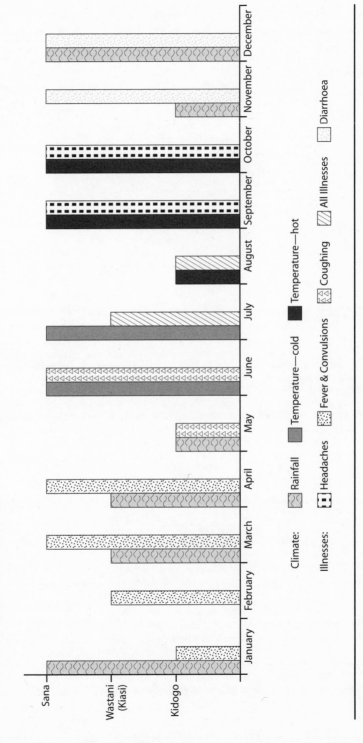

FIGURE 5

Seasonal Calendar for Illnesses and Climate in Asanje, Tanzania (Number of Participants/Informants = 16)

and Box 17). Here, the Lunar calendar traditionally used by the Gogo was equated roughly to the Gregorian (European) calendar. The labels on the vertical axis signify a little *(kidogo)*, medium/average *(wastani/kiasi)*, and a lot *(sana)* in *Kiswahili*. Participants were asked to concentrate on illnesses that affected children over the past year. The information provided included adult illnesses as well, and it was suggested that the same climatic and illness pattern occurred most years.

A seasonal calendar, stored on a flip-chart or other type of paper, such as the one on Figure 5 which can be found in the Dodoma hygiene evaluation study report, can serve as a document that can be used for reference and/or monitoring purposes.

BOX 17

Extracts of Notes from Discussions of a Seasonal Calendar

From Asanje Village, Tanzania

In Asanje village, seasonal calendars for activities, diseases, and climate were prepared in the same session. The participants included twelve women and nine men who began by discussing the common illnesses. The first illness mentioned was *degedege* which strictly speaking refers to convulsions. The term is commonly used for malaria. However, the term *homa*, fever, was also used in the discussion to refer to malaria. Both fever and convulsions were associated with the wet season. Participants agreed that degedege is a common illness during the months of January to April. There is little of it (that is, a few people have it, mainly children) in January; more in February (average numbers of people); but a lot in March and April (almost all young children and several adults suffer from it). The traditional doctor mentioned that he had treated many people for degedege in the past few months. The women participants recalled the children who had died from degedege in recent months, but they did not mention any adults...

The amount of rainfall was high in January, very little in February, average in March and April, and little in May...

When asked why the *shamba* was extended after planting and not before, the participants explained that it was for safety reasons. If the shamba is very close to the bush, it is more difficult for the farmer to protect his crop from raids by wild animals such as baboons and wild boar without him/herself risking attacks by other wild animals including hyenas, leopards and cheetahs. The men reported that at the time of this study, they were having to spend all night outdoors guarding their shambas from wild boar...

The temperature was said to be a little hot in August, but very hot in September and October. In September and October most adults (particularly women) suffered from headaches. This was said to be the main illness which affected large numbers of people. Headaches were caused by walking long distances (to Babayu and Maya Maya) to fetch water every day. Women carried water on their heads while men, who usually helped to fetch water during these two months, were said to use wheelbarrows or bicycles, if available. The participants discussed and agreed that many people suffered from diarrhoea in November and December when the rains began.

Gender Roles/Tasks Analysis

Investigating gender issues particularly in relation to task allocation and resource management is important for understanding the context in which hygiene practices occur. One of the ways to explore this with participants is to use pictures depicting many of the activities observed locally. Participants should discuss these and arrive at a consensus as to whether each task depicted is performed by men, women, or both.

The same principle can be applied to a set of pictures showing locally produced and used resources and asking which ones are controlled by men, which by women, and which by both men and women.

Purpose

■ To find out which activities or tasks are acceptable for men, which are assigned to women, and which are acceptable for both men and women in the local culture, and why.

■ To find out how existing resources are shared between men and women in the society, which resources are managed and/or owned by men, by women, or by both.

Materials

Have a set of fifteen to twenty-five cards (pictures mounted on thick paper or card board) showing relevant activities or tasks that are common in the study site, such as fetching water, building latrines, cleaning latrines, feeding children, tilling the land, and so on, for investigating gender-specific activities and tasks; have about the same number of pictures/cards showing commonly used resources such as money, livestock, household goods, and so on for investigating the type of resources for which men and women have access and control. Have three pictures/cards depicting a local adult man, an adult woman, and a man and woman together. The pictures can be drawn by local artists or borrowed from existing locally prepared illustrated booklets, or sets of photographs which may be enlarged and photocopied for this purpose. It is important that the cards show local settings and practices. Label each card with a number so you can refer to it when recording people's comments.

Procedure

The following guidelines may be helpful to the facilitator:

■ Introduce yourself and indicate why the meeting is taking place. Speak clearly, using the local language.

■ Ask participants whether the pictures show familiar scenes and whether the tasks shown are commonly undertaken by men, women, or both, and why. When investigating resource allocation and management, ask whether the resources shown are common and who normally controls or manages them, men, women or both, and why.

■ If it is useful (e.g., to enable participants to talk more freely, or to find opinions of different sections of the study population) divide participants into smaller groups, for example, according to gender, or age.

■ Hand out the cards and ask participants to pass them around, taking time to look at them closely, then discuss each card.

■ Listen and learn.

■ Ask the group to decide which category each card fits into: good, bad, or in-between. Remind them that they can use the in-between option if the pictures are unclear, or if the group has not agreed whether the practice is good or bad.

■ Take notes on what people say (including the final decision, and how many people attended), but do not interfere with the discussion.

Management, Review, and Use of Information

The following procedures will help you process the information obtained systematically:

■ Write up your notes. Describe the participants/samples and summarize what each group said about the cards. List the main points made and issues raised in the discussion, areas of disagreement, and any unexpected ideas that were suggested. This information will indicate what participants believe is the job, responsibility, or property of a man or a woman, and what is shared by both man and woman, but it does not prove anything. It can be a starting point for more investigation using other methods such as observation, interviewing, and focus group discussion of the main issues raised.

■ List the pictures by number and collate each group's comments on each picture.

■ Review the comments made by each group and identify common views and beliefs. Define specific questions for further investigation.

■ Prepare reduced copies of each picture used to put in your study report alongside your summaries of the comments made. These may be placed in an annex/appendix to the main body of your report form and Box 18).

Appraisal of the Methods and Tools

Each of the methods and tools listed were appraised on the basis of our experiences of their use in the context of water supply, sanitation, and health/hygiene education projects, in five different sites in Asia and East Africa during the development and field testing of this handbook. The practical constraints faced by project personnel are reflected, for instance, where the need for well trained and skilled investigators/discussion facilitators is mentioned under limitations, it relates to the scarcity of such human resources in the average project setting.

It is important to note that many of the methods and tools described have uses that go well beyond the purposes of investigation and analysis. In particular, those originating from participatory approaches have sustainable educational value because they arouse people's awareness of their own hygiene practices and other issues in the context in which they live. The effect of their awareness and reflection upon the results of investigation can be long-lasting, providing a good foundation for hygiene/health promotion activities (see Chapter 7 for the uses of information in project implementation).

BOX   18
Comments on the Gender Task Pictures on Plate 1

From Afghanistan and Ethiopia

Picture 1
  (a) "This is a man's job, but a woman could do it as well—if she was trained in the repairing of pipes and pumps." (Ethiopia, mixed group of men and women in a small town)

  (b) "This is usually done by men, but we can do it as well, if we are trained." (Afghanistan, group of women in a village)

Picture 2
  (a) "Both men and women teach, at schools, clinics and health centres." (Ethiopia, mixed group of men and women in a small town)

  (b) "Yes, we have women teachers, but this is not the way it is done here...Men and women are taught separately. Also, you can't have adults and children in the same class, and a woman does not teach outdoors, only indoors." (Afghanistan, group of women in a village)

PLATE 1

Pictures Used in Gender Task Analysis in Ethopia (1994) and Afghanistan (1996)

Picture 1

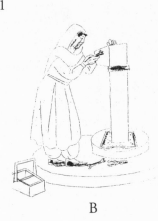

A   B

Picture 2

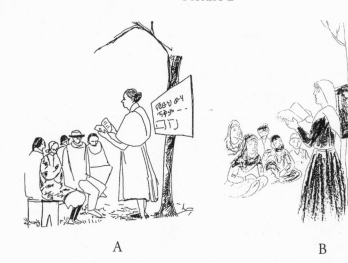

A   B

T A B L E 3

Strengths and Limitations of the Methods and Tools Described in Chapter 5

Method/Tool	Strengths	Limitations
Healthwalk	+ Helps investigators to get a general feel of the study site and people (involves all their senses) in a short period of time. + Allows investigators to conduct spot-check observations, to get known by members of the study population, to recruit participants for group discussions and to identify key-informants relatively quickly and easily. + Allows investigators to explore relevant issues, to identify possible leads of inquiry and/or to formulate hypotheses.	▪ May lead to wrong first impressions and important issues may be overlooked if investigators are not alert, do not have the right attitudes and/or are inadequately trained. ▪ May need to be done repeatedly to cover different times of day or different seasons, and thus require considerable time and other resources (especially if access to the study site is difficult) for the identification of relevant issues and revising choice of methods and tools. This may be overcome by extending the period of preplanning to include the conduct of healthwalks in the study site(s).
Structured (Spot-Check) Observations	+ Provides systematic information which can be quantified. + Allows the collection of relatively accurate information (compared to reported information) unobtrusively and so are good for crosschecking information (triangulation).	▪ Requires skilled and disciplined investigators to manage the information/field notes, to analyze and document findings. ▪ Does not allow feedback, or enhance active participation by members of the study population.
Key-Informant Interviews	+ Allows investigators to gain indepth knowledge of the subject under study. + Provides rich sets of information (with answers to the *why* questions) which can be used for exploring certain issues further, crosschecking/triangulation purposes and for the interpretation of findings. + Relatively easy to document findings, e.g., without investing in visual aids.	▪ May introduce bias to the study, if the number of key-informants is limited and/or not representative of more than one section of the study population. ▪ Requires prolonged engagement with the key-informant and thus more time, unless investigators are already well known to informants. ▪ Requires time and skills to manage and review information from detailed field notes.

TABLE 3
Strengths and Limitations of the Methods and Tools Described in Chapter 5 (continued)

Method/Tool	Strengths	Limitations
Historyline	+ Good for establishing or improving rapport with the study population by demonstrating that their version of local history is valued. + Useful for finding out how local people see themselves, which historical events and/or personalities are important to them, and why. + The results can be easily presented to a larger meeting of study participants for confirmation or correction.	- Information obtained requires crosschecking with documentary sources, if available, and thus requires more time for analysis.
Community Mapping	+ Quick, effective, inexpensive, and accurate way of gathering basic information. + Allows study participants to engage in investigative and analytical processes, increasing their level of participation awareness of the issues at hand. + The map can be easily presented to a larger meeting of study participants for confirmation or correction. + Provides project personnel and study participants an easily accessible visual documentation which can serve as a record in itself and as a tool for monitoring progress. + Heightens study participants' awareness of and reflections on their situation.	- Requires well-trained, skilled facilitator(s) and note-taker(s).

TABLE 3

Strengths and Limitations of the Methods and Tools Described in Chapter 5 (continued)

Method/Tool	Strengths	Limitations
Seasonal Calendar	✦ Useful for articulating and systematically documenting local knowledge. ✦ Provides insight into local patterns of climate, disease and subsistence activities and the reasons behind certain practices (some of which may be water/sanitation-related). ✦ The results can be easily presented to a larger meeting of study participants for confirmation or correction. ✦ Heightens study participants' awareness of and reflections on their situation.	▪ Requires skilled facilitators. ▪ Information obtained requires crosschecking with documentary sources, if available, and thus may require additional time for analysis and interpretation.
Gender Roles Analysis	✦ Quick and effective for exploring gender issues with (pictorial) reference to gender-specific roles and management of resources in a given culture. ✦ Provides investigators with insight into the role of women, children, and men in preserving existing hygiene practices. ✦ Increases awareness of gender issues among study participants—a step towards instigating change where it may be necessary.	▪ Requires time and special skills to prepare, pretest, and subsequently modify the pictures. ▪ Requires skilled facilitators. ▪ Difficult to document results by using words (text) only, thus costly (in terms of time and money) to document.

6

Investigating Hygiene Practices

- *Three-Pile Sorting*
- *Pocket Chart*
- *Semi-Structured (Informal) Interviews*
- *Focus Group Discussion*
- *Appraisal of the Methods and Tools*

The following methods and tools have been field tested for investigating specific clusters of hygiene practices. Each one can be adapted or modified for specific settings whenever necessary. You may also want to include additional methods and tools from your particular training and experience, provided that they fulfil the selection criteria outlined in Chapter 5 (see Diagram 3).

Three-Pile Sorting

This method derives from the Promotion of the Role of Women in Water and Environmental Sanitation Services (PROWWESS) participatory approach (Srinivasan, 1990). Participants are given a set of drawings showing situations related to defecation, protection of water sources, water use and personal hygiene, food hygiene, corralling of domestic animals, and so on. Participants are then asked to discuss each drawing as a group and to arrive at a consensus as to whether it is good, bad, or in-between, and to explain why. Three-pile sorting operates in the same way as gender roles/tasks analysis, the only difference being that the three piles consist of good, bad, and in-between, instead of man, woman, and both.

Purpose

■ To break down barriers and establish good communication. For this reason, it is a good tool to use at the beginning of fieldwork.

■ To introduce sensitive/personal topics for discussion such as latrine use and personal cleanliness at the early stages of enquiry.

Materials

A set of twelve to sixteen cards (pictures mounted on thick paper or card board) showing activities related to sanitation and water-related hygiene should be used. The drawings can be drawn by local artists or adapted from health-related illustrated handbooks. It is important that the cards show local settings and practices. Each of the situations depicted should include at least one activity and/or feature that relates to one or more of the five clusters of hygiene practices (see, for instance, Plate 2).

The exact content of the drawings will depend on the hygiene practices you have decided to focus on, and on the materials available. Situations that are not hygiene-related but may be of crucial interest to the smooth running of your project, such as issues of user participation or operation and maintenance, may also be included. Label each card with a number so that you can refer to the number when writing down people's comments.

Procedure

The following guidelines may be helpful to the facilitator:

■ Introduce yourself and indicate why the meeting is taking place. Speak clearly, using the local language.

■ Ask participants whether the pictures show familiar scenes and whether the practices shown are good or bad, and why.

■ If it is useful (e.g., to enable participants to talk more freely, or to find opinions of different sections of the study population) divide participants into smaller groups, for example, according to gender or age.

■ Hand out the cards and ask participants to pass them around, taking time to look at them closely, then discuss each card.

■ Listen and learn.

■ Ask the group to decide which category each card fits into: good, bad, or in-between. Remind them that they can use the in-between option

PLATE 2
Pictures Used for Three Pile Sorting in India (1996)

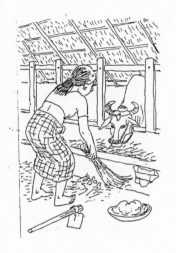

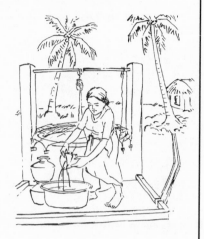

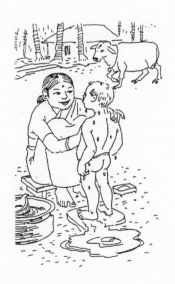

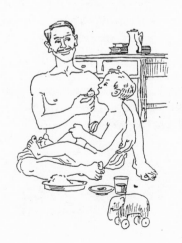

if the pictures are unclear, or if the group has not agreed whether the practice is good or bad.

■ Take notes on what people say (including the final decision, and how many people attended), but do not interfere with the discussion.

Management, Review, and Use of Information

■ Write up your notes. Describe the participants/samples and summarize what each group said about the cards (see Box 19 for an example of sample description). List the main points made and issues raised in the discussion, areas of disagreement, and any unexpected ideas that were suggested.

This information will indicate what participants believe is good or bad hygiene practice, and what they decide is in-between, but it does not prove anything. It can be a starting point for more investigation using other methods such as observation, interviewing, and focus group discussion of the main issues of disagreement.

■ List the pictures by number and collate each group's comments with each picture.

■ Review the comments made by each group and identify common views and beliefs, as well as unexpected issues raised which may be unrelated to hygiene practices. For example, the picture on Plate 3 (the same picture translated to relate to two different ethnic and cultural groups) generated animated discussions of family planning with particular reference to the responsibilities of the man (see Box 20). Define specific questions for further investigation.

BOX 19

Three-Pile Sorting—Sample Description Examples from Two Tanzanian Villages

Village 1		Village 2	
Group	Number	Group	Number
First group of village notables	13	Wanaume maarufu, influential men	10
Second group of village notables	9	Wanawake maarufu, influential women	8
School boys	11	Wanawake, ordinary women (mixed age)	12
School girls	10	Wanafunzi wavulana, school boys	18
Young men	20	Wanafunzi wasichana, school girls	11
		Vijana, young men	23

PLATE 3

One of the Three Pile Sorting Cards Used in Tanzania (1994)

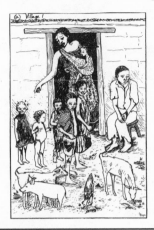 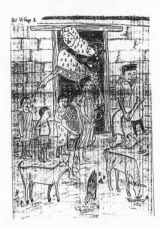

BOX 20

Summary of Comments on the Picture Shown in Plate 3

From Dodoma Region, Tanzania

Village 1

"Very bad. This is bad family planning. The man looks confused. They must be very poor, because one of the children has no clothes on. The woman has no time to clean the surroundings. She has too many children. It is also bad to have the animals everywhere." (First group of village notables)

"Bad and common in this village. The man loves his wife too much—there are many like him who keep making their wives pregnant. One of the children has an infected scalp which is why flies are attracted to her head. It is bad to leave a child naked, and the surroundings are not clean." (Second group of village notables)

"Bad because the children are dirty—one of them has scalp infection which is why she is attracting flies. All of the children look thin and their father has no shoes. Such situations are common here." (Group of young men.)

Village 2

"In-between. The man has no shoes nor do his children. This is bad. One of the girls has attracted flies by not washing her face. It is good that the mother is telling her off. The other children have washed their faces which is why there are no flies near them." [No mention of the man.] (Group of influential men)

"Bad, because the woman has too many children. She has no time to look after them all. [This was followed by a long discussion of family planning.] (Group of influential women)

"Bad, because there is no child spacing here. The man is bad, he has been forcing the woman to conceive frequently. he should use "socks." [Some of them started singing the popular song, "You better put socks on," composed and sung by a Doctor Remy Ongala.] We have many men like this one in our village, if you want, we can show them to you. The environment is not clean." (Group of young men)

FIGURE 6

Pictures Used in a Pocket Chart to Investigate Water Uses According to Source, Showing the Number of Votes (Kenya, 1993)

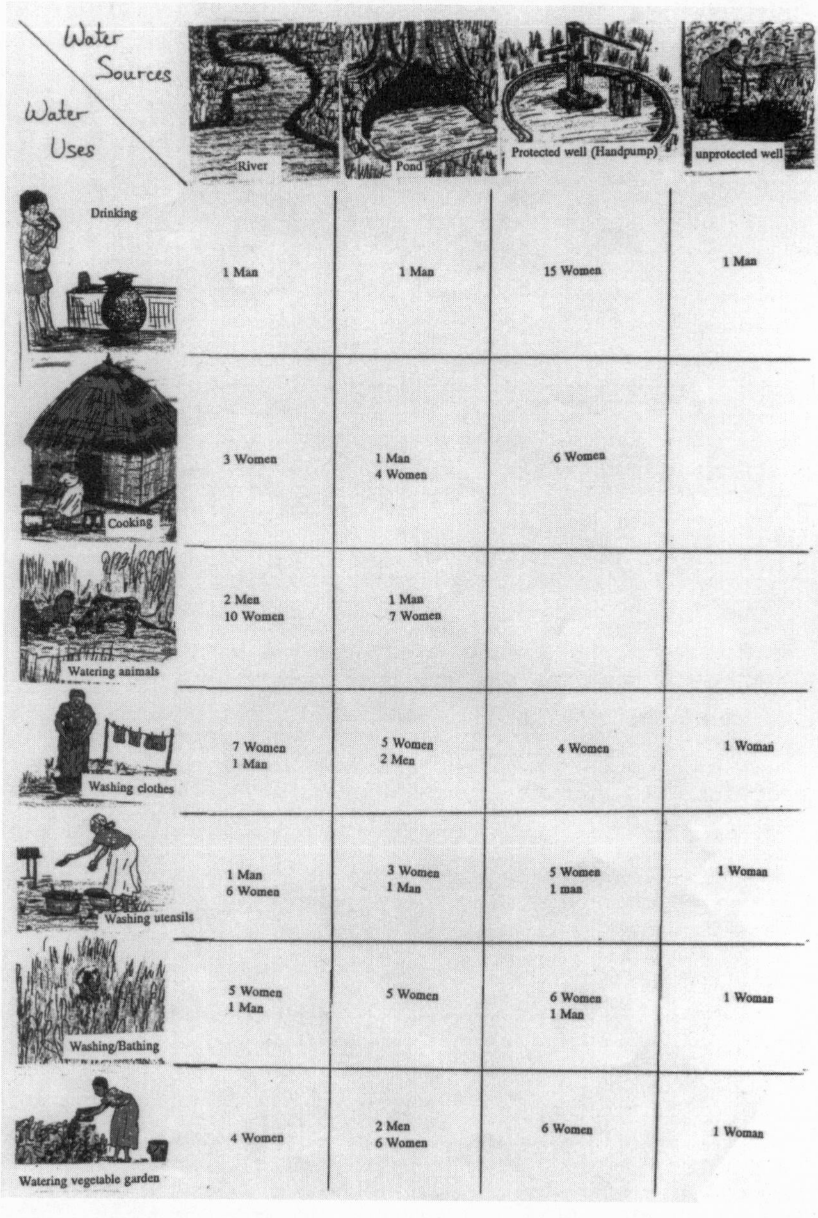

Water Sources / Water Uses	River	Pond	Protected well (Handpump)	unprotected well
Drinking	1 Man	1 Man	15 Women	1 Man
Cooking	3 Women	1 Man 4 Women	6 Women	
Watering animals	2 Men 10 Women	1 Man 7 Women		
Washing clothes	7 Women 1 Man	5 Women 2 Men	4 Women	1 Woman
Washing utensils	1 Man 6 Women	3 Women 1 Man	5 Women 1 man	1 Woman
Washing/Bathing	5 Women 1 Man	5 Women	6 Women 1 Man	1 Woman
Watering vegetable garden	4 Women	2 Men 6 Women	6 Women	1 Woman

■ Prepare reduced copies of each picture used to put in your study report along with your summaries of the comments made. These may be placed in an annex/appendix to the main body of your report for reference in order to save space and to facilitate easy reading (see Plate 3 and Box 20).

Pocket Chart

This tool derives from PROWWESS, and can be used in many different ways depending on the topic of investigation and the type of information required.

Purpose

■ To investigate which water source is used for what purpose, or who uses which defecation site and to find out the reasons why. For example, in one study the pocket chart was used for collecting and tabulating data on water sources in relation to water uses. In another study it was used for investigating choice of defecation sites (courtyard, traditional latrine, SANPLAT latrine, VIP latrine, bush) according to different members of a household—child, woman, man, senior man, senior woman (See Figure 6).

BOX 21
Extracts from Pocket Chart Discussion Notes

From a Village in Western Kenya

When the study team announced the voting results the participants reviewed and discussed the results. Of a total of twenty participants (seventeen women, three men), the majority, fifteen women indicated that they fetched water for drinking from the handpump. This was because they perceived that water to be clean and the source was convenient as most of them lived near the borehole. When it came to fetching water for other uses, however, the handpump was far less popular. It is clear, therefore, that these women used their rational decision making skills when choosing water sources.

The review session allowed participants to confirm and/or question the votes: one young man questioned the trustworthiness of the number of votes relating to the use of handpump water for watering the vegetable garden. He stated that he did not believe that the six women were telling the truth. "How do these women manage to have enough of that water to use for watering their garden?" he asked. Others agreed with him as they knew that, on any one day, each household was allowed to collect only two buckets of water from the handpump. The women discussed this question before one of them explained that besides drinking, they were using water from the handpump for other purposes, such as washing utensils before "throwing it out on the garden." This was a simple case of water recycling, and an example of the rational management of a scarce resource.

Materials

A wide variety of materials may be used for making the pocket chart. The main components include a set of pictures for each variable (e.g., depicting a water source or a water use); material on which these pictures are placed (a wall, a piece of canvas or other strong material, or the ground); pieces of paper/card, pebbles or beads for "voting," indicating variables selected; pockets or other receptacles in which the voting cards or pebbles or beads are put.

Procedure

- Introduce yourself, your team, and explain the purpose of the meeting clearly in the local language.

- Introduce the pocket chart by showing it to the participants and describe the materials of which it is made.

- Ask the participants to pass the pictures around and to discuss what is depicted. Listen and learn.

- Arrive at a consensus with the participants on what each picture depicts. You must make sure that any ambiguity in the participants' minds about what each picture depicts is fully discussed and clarified so that it is clear to each participant what the variables are.

- Ask participants whether they would like to add any other variables that may have been left out. If the answer is yes, find a picture or symbol to depict each additional variable (if the study team includes an artist, this may be prepared on the spot and passed around to the participants for their approval.

- Start with blank pockets, and explain the voting procedure.

- Conduct a demonstration—mock voting in the open.

- Distribute voting cards—assign a different colour for each gender and/or age group, if necessary.

- Cover the pockets, and turn the pocket chart around so that people can vote privately by secret balloting, and start the voting process using one variable at a time.

- Reveal the results to the participants before proceeding to the next variable.

- Record the number of votes in each pocket.

■ Review/discuss the results with the participants.

Management, Review, and Use of Information

■ Write up your notes from the discussion that took place during the use of the pocket chart.

■ Keep the tabulated voting results and prepare a chart showing the pictures or description of them in words and the number of votes as shown in Figure 6 (see Box 21 for an example of pocket chart discussion notes).

Semi-Structured (Informal) Interviews

The semi-structured interviewing method is also part of the standard anthropological investigative approach.

Purpose

■ To investigate general as well as specific issues by asking questions informally but systematically.

■ To find out which hygiene practices are considered ideal or acceptable, and why.

Tool

A written interview schedule should be prepared for the interviewer to study beforehand. This involves specific training of the study team to enable them to learn or improve their interviewing techniques, discussions of possible lines of questioning, modifications of the question lines, translation of agreed questions into the local language(s), and back-translating from the local language into English in order to check that the intended meaning is conveyed. A semi-structured interview schedule (see the Worksheet 2 for an example) is often used prior to the conduct of interviews rather than during the actual interviews.

Procedure

■ Study your semi-structured interview schedule well in advance to familiarize yourself with the scope of the questions and the question lines selected. You can make your own brief set of notes to remind you of the question lines developed and the topics covered. Rehearse your question lines in the presence of others in your team and ask them to give you their constructive criticism (see Chapter 3).

■ If possible, have another member of your study team accompany you to the interviewee's home and sit through the interview as a note-taker.

■ Introduce yourself, the note-taker, and any other members of the study team present (e.g., the observer); establish good rapport with the interviewee and his/her family (see the Introduction to Chapter 3).

■ Listen carefully and use common sense, however well you may have memorized or studied the interview schedule beforehand. For example, do not ask the respondent whether her children are old enough to use a latrine if she has already told you that she has no children.

■ Avoid asking leading questions.

■ Use prompts and probes sensitively.

■ Draw the interview to a close by thanking your interviewee and any others who have assisted you.

Management, Review, and Use of Information

At the end of each day of interviewing, try to find time to write up the interview notes as a team. The notes jotted down during the interview might be very brief, but now these need to be expanded and annotated. You can expand the notes by adding in detail what you did not have time to write down but now recall, and you can annotate by writing your own ideas—relevant questions, importance of findings, themes, and so on— on the notes. It can be useful to have wide margins for your notes, or to write on one side of the page only, using the opposite page for comments and additional information.

Information obtained by interviews is usually analyzed by systems of categorizing, indexing, and filing to facilitate its management and analysis. For example, a separate file or index can be kept for each cluster or sub-cluster of hygiene practices, or for each category of information about the local context. Special computer software packages are now available for use in textual data analysis, however, a simple word-processing package, if available, can also make the job of filing and indexing qualitative information easier and faster. See Box 22 for an example of how interview and observation data can be recorded, before they are reviewed by the study team.

Worksheet 2
An Example of a Semi-Structured Interview Guide

Name:

Village/Town/City/Camp/Zone/Section:

1. Greetings (for example, "Good morning/afternoon; How are you and how are the children? Other members of the family? etc.)

*2. How many children do you have?

Girls: _____   Boys: _____
Name   Age   Name   Age

3. Are the children able to use the latrine on their own?

4. If not, where do they defecate?

5. How do you dispose of the faeces?

6. Who else uses the latrine?

7. Do you use the latrine?

8. If not, why not?

9. Do you think young children's faeces are harmful in any way?

10. Why?

*   This may be a sensitive question in many cultures although we did not find any problem posing it after the preceding question (expressing interest in the children's well-being). An alternative may be, "*Tell me about your children.*"

11. Have the children had diarrhoea in the last two or three days?

12. What caused it?

13. How did you treat it?

14. Who else has suffered from diarrhoea in the last two or three days?

15. How was it treated?

16. Where do you get your water from?

17. How much? How often?

18. What is it used for?

19. Do you treat water before drinking or other use
    (a) by filtering
    (b) by allowing it to settle
    (c) by pouring ash in and allowing it to settle
    (d) by boiling
    (e) by other means?

20. Do you pay for water? How much?

21. When do you wash your hands with soap/ash/other local soap alternative?

22. Why? If not, why not?

BOX 22

Extract from Informal Interview and Observation Notes/Summaries

From Asanje Village, Tanzania

Interview 1—Christina (a pseudonym is used to protect the identity of the respondent)

Around ten o'clock in the morning, we saw Christina, a young mother working in a *shamba*. Upon greeting her, we discovered that her house was very close. We made it clear that we were interested in chatting with her a bit longer so she invited us to stop over at her house.

Christina has four children ages twelve (a girl), nine (a girl), six years, and an infant of eighteen months. Christina said that everyone is able to use the latrine except her youngest child. This infant normally defecates outside the house. Christina disposes of the child's faeces in the latrine. [The study team recalled that during the healthwalk they conducted on the previous day they had seen Christina. She was carrying child's faeces on a hoe and scattering it on the *shamba* using a bunch of leaves to sweep it off the hoe.] Christina also said that everyone else in her household uses the latrine. When asked whether she thought children's faeces were harmful in any way, Christina said that children's faeces have an offensive smell and they cause diseases. Christina reported that both her six year old and the eighteen month old children had diarrhoea a few days ago. It was caused by *degedege*, convulsions (often associated with malaria). She explained that the convulsions had caused "foaming in the mouth," and "the foams that did not appear in the mouth turned into diarrhoea."

Christina fetches water from the seasonal spring in the mornings, one bucket (twenty liter capacity) and her children fetch the same amount in the afternoons. She uses that water for drinking, cooking, and washing utensils. She washes clothes at the water source. She stores drinking water in a pot without a cover, and everyone in her household uses the same *kipeyo* (an oval-shaped bowl made of calabash, used both for scooping water out of the hand-dug wells and for drinking). Christina has paid her contribution (400 Shillings for a year) to the village water fund. Christina reported that she washes her hands first thing in the morning, before cooking, and before and after eating. She explained that everyone in her family washes hands in the same bowl of water (without soap) before eating. Christina stores food (milk and maize flour) in a *kangambwa*, a hanging pot or calabash.

Spot-check observations showed that the compound had been swept clean. The latrine superstructure consisted of a short mud wall. The latrine floor was swept clean and ashes were sprinkled around the hole.

Focus Group Discussion

This method derives from market research strategies in which theories of social psychology and communication were applied and later incorporated into social sciences research methods. A special manual for the use of focus group discussions in health research is now available (see Dawson, Manderson and Tallo, 1993).

In a focus group discussion, people from similar backgrounds or experiences (e.g., mothers, young married men, birth attendants/mid-wives) are brought together to discuss a specific topic of interest to the investigator(s). Homogeneous samples are preferred because mixing age/

gender groups may inhibit some people, especially women, from expressing their views.

Purpose

- To explore the range of opinions/views on a topic of interest.

- To collect a wide variety of local terms and expressions used to describe a disease (e.g., diarrhoea) or an act (e.g., defecation).

- To explore meanings of survey findings that cannot be explained statistically.

Materials

A range of materials including tape recorders, if appropriate, and pictures to introduce topics for discussion, can be used. Recording the discussion on tape has the advantage of being able to play it back and pick up salient points after the discussion is over. The disadvantage is that transcribing from tape takes a long time—it can take up to five hours to transcribe an hour's tape recording of a focus group discussion plus another couple of hours to listen to the tape again and check the transcription for accuracy. Even then important points may be missed if the tape recording is not accompanied by detailed notes on who the participants were, the order in which they spoke, and the non-verbal language which accompanied what was said. If the discussion took place in a language not understood by the investigator(s), translation can mean added time and financial costs. See Box 23 for an example of notes transcribed from a focus group discussion held with committee members of a *Harambé*, a self-help, rainwater harvesting project in Kenya (*P* signifies participants whose names were coded by the letters of the alphabet and *M* stands for the discussion moderator. The discussion was conducted in *Kiswahili*).

Procedure

- Identify suitable discussion participants and invite a small group to a meeting at an agreed place and time. The ideal number of participants is six to eight, but be flexible about numbers—do not turn away participants after they had arrived at the meeting and do not pressure people to come to the meeting. Study the Focus Group Manual for detailed guidance (see also Chapter 3).

BOX 23

Extract of Notes from a Focus Group Discussion

Transcribed and Literally Translated from Kiswahili into English

From a Village in Kenya

P(A): Even what that one has said is higher (important) that is what we have heard, that one continues and the goodness of it is this. It has helped us in the health of our children.

M: Say according to the way you see. Don't say according to the way you think we would like to hear. Now you yourself since you got that tank, how do you see it has helped? You have a tank at home, how has it helped?

P(A): It has helped us very much because I can see when we drink water there are no diseases like stomachaches. It has helped very much and me, I can see when you drink other water it is not as good as the one in the tank.

M: And do you use this water for cooking?

P(A): Yes.

M: Does it help you and you don't have to fetch water in the mornings, so you don't get tired?

P(F): Yes we don't get tired these days, because when there were no tanks we had to go with jericans to the river, but, now, I can see these days I just sit and then I just fetch water and come to cook and help to wash clothes. These days I don't go to the river. Yes, and even the cows and calves they drink at home. Yes, it has helped very much.

P(C): It has taken money.

P(B): Yes, that has taken our money. (Laughter) We can see that others cannot help build. Because they come to our home to beg for good water for drinking. But we see if they help build another if we get some little help, because others cannot build. (interruption) Yes, so that we can build.

M: Is there anything you want to say about the sanitation?

P(H): Yes, concerning matters about latrines? Yes there I could say this is something we need very much. Latrines for use, because many people, despite many people trying to dig latrines and build, me, I see that they make them in the proper way...You find people have dug holes (for the latrines) but the next year the latrine has collapsed and cannot be used...Something that will be needed in this matter of sanitation is these people, technicians, those who know how to build latrines, like those technicians of AMREF. We have seen the ones they have built in schools and now even people are waiting anxiously...People should go on building latrines and they should be helped to build those ones of now (modern ones). The ones they can use nicely and for a long time. I was saying the idea of the water tanks is good rather than for people to wait for rain water to go down the stream, sweeping all the dirt then go for it, they would rather collect it from the roofs, so I must say this water tanks have assisted a lot. Yeah, for those who have, they see the sense and importance of it. And for those who don't have, very many are more than willing to build these water tanks. Yes.

M: Do you want to say something on sanitation? Talk in Kiswahili.

P(A): For the truth, AMREF has really tried very much because they have built latrines in the schools. There is where the students learn and it would be useful so much, if sanitation is followed. Now I can see even the way we have succeeded in building latrines in schools even now I can say, I wish we could go to the communities and build latrines if we can because we have succeeded in schools. Since latrines have been made in schools, we have seen many diseases have decreased. Diseases like tapeworms have decreased in hospitals. Now, I would like, if AMREF would continue to build latrines for people. We can take at least one person from every village. Me, I think, on matters concerning sanitation that is all.

■ Be mentally prepared for the session; you will need to remain alert to be able to observe, listen, and keep the discussion on track for a period of one to two hours.

■ Make sure you arrive at the agreed place before the participants, and be ready to greet them.

■ Maintain a neutral attitude and appearance, and do not start talking about the topic of interest before the official opening of the group discussion.

■ Begin by introducing yourself and your team (even if the participants have already met them individually), and ask participants to introduce themselves.

■ Explain clearly that the purpose of the discussion is to find out what people think about the practices or activities depicted by the pictures. Tell them that you are not looking for any right or wrong answer but that you want to learn what each participant's views are. It must be made clear to all participants that their views will be valued.

■ Bring the discussion to a close when you feel the topic has been exhausted, and do not let the group discussion degenerate into smaller discussions. Be sincere in expressing your thanks to the participants for their contributions. Refreshments may be served at the end of the meeting as a way of thanking the participants and maintaining good rapport with them.

Management, Review, and Use of Information

The Focus Group Manual (Dawson, Manderson and Tallo, 1993) suggests that all discussion be transcribed. If you decide to use a tape recorder, you may prefer to transcribe parts of the discussion only to save time. In this case, listen carefully to the tape at least once, and mark down the sections that you wish to have transcribed, using the counter and summarize the information. Once you have a transcript before you, have checked it with the tape, and made any necessary corrections, then mark up the text.

We have found it practical for the intended users of this handbook to use a modified form of focus group discussion in which pictures (often selected from the sets prepared for three-pile sorting or gender tasks and resources analysis) are used to introduce often sensitive topics such as defecation behaviour and associated hygiene practices. Using pictures helped to stimulate discussion of specific issues very quickly. Without pictures, people tend to feel that they have to make a set speech every time they intervene, and they tend to cover more than one topic at a time (as can be seen in Box 23).

Study team members take the roles of a discussion facilitator/moderator, a note-taker, and an observer. All three would then meet afterwards to write up comprehensive notes, including the facilitator's impressions, the observer's notes, and the note-taker's detailed notes.

Appraisal of the Methods and Tools

The general rule is that no single method and/or tool on its own is perfect for assessing hygiene practices. One may be good for one purpose (for example, gathering information in a short period of time) while another may be good for another purpose (for example, obtaining detailed and extensive indepth information). Given that it is desirable, if not necessary, to use more than one method and/or tool in your study, decisions about which ones to select may be easier once you have consulted our appraisal of individual methods and tools from a predominantly practical perspective. Weighing the strengths and limitations of each method and tool is essential in deciding which combination(s) of methods and tools to use (see Table 4).

TABLE 4

Strengths and Limitations of the Methods and Tools Described in Chapter 6

Method/Tool	Strengths	Limitations
Three-Pile Sorting	✦ Good for breaking the ice and initiating discussion on sensitive topics, particularly when investigators' knowledge of the local culture and language(s) are limited (for instance, explicit pictures of open defecation will introduce the topic of discussion more directly and effectively than words can). ✦ Effective for finding out which hygiene behaviours and activities are locally considered to be good, bad, or in-between and more importantly, *why*. ✦ Allows study participants to engage in investigative and analytical processes which will increase their awareness of their own hygiene practices—a step towards instigating change where it may be necessary.	▪ Requires time and special skills to prepare, pretest, and subsequently modify the pictures. ▪ Requires well-trained and skilled facilitator(s). ▪ Difficult to document results by using words (text) only, thus costly (in terms of time and money) to document.
Pocket Chart	✦ Relatively quick and effective way of gathering quantifiable information and interpreting it quickly and reliably. ✦ Allows study participants to engage in investigative and analytical processes which will increase their awareness of their own hygiene practices—a step towards instigating change where it may be necessary. ✦ Easy to document results.	▪ Requires time and special skills to prepare, pretest, and subsequently modify the pictures. ▪ Requires well-trained and skilled facilitator(s). ▪ Requires time and patience/motivation from study participants, particularly if the number of variables involved exceeds three or four. ▪ Difficult to conduct effectively with large groups (more than twenty people).

TABLE 4

Strengths and Limitations of the Methods and Tools Described in Chapter 6 (continued)

Method/Tool	Strengths	Limitations
Semi-Structured Interviews	+ Allows investigators to gain indepth knowledge of the subject under study. + Relatively easy to document findings, e.g., without investing in visual aids.	▪ Requires highly skilled and/or trained investigators, interviewers, and note-takers. ▪ May be intrusive to study participants, especially if hurriedly done and/or with little tact. ▪ Presents difficulty for interviewers if they are project personnel who are seen by the study population more as teachers/experts than as learners—respondents may give all the "right answers" which may not reflect their own practices, or may demand that the interviewer(s) gives them answers to difficult questions as she/he is an expert anyway. ▪ Requires considerable amounts of time and energy for information management and review.
Focus Group Discussions	+ Useful for gauging the range of opinions and beliefs on the topic of enquiry. + Useful for exploring issues for investigation at the outset of a study and/or for interpreting data obtained by other methods (including quantitative surveys) in the final stages of a study. + Easily modifiable to facilitate its use, e.g., by using pictures to introduce topics for discussion and for stimulating/maintaining a lively discussion.	▪ Information obtained cannot stand on its own, i.e., it needs to be complemented by survey data, to show the distribution of opinions and beliefs uncovered. ▪ Presents difficulties in information management and review, particularly if tape-recorders are used. ▪ If more than one language is in use, translation can mean added time and financial costs.

7

Analysis, Presentation, and Implementation of Findings

- *Stages of Analysis and Interpretation of Findings*
- *Establishing the Trustworthiness of Information*
- *Presentation of Findings*
- *Implementation of Findings*

By the time you finish using the methods and tools you have selected for your study, you will have several sets of information organized and stored in notebooks, files, and index cards according to chronological order or by method/tool used, or both. This chapter deals with the processes of conducting overall analysis of all the information gathered and reviewed; checking its trustworthiness by triangulation; interpreting or making sense of findings; presentation and use of findings. As documentation is one of the most important outputs of a hygiene evaluation study, we shall demonstrate how investigation and analysis link up to report writing in practical terms.

Stages of Analysis and Interpretation of Findings

There are four main stages in the analysis and interpretation of qualitative information. These are discussed in more detail in several text books including Patton (1986, 1990), Miles and Huberman (1994), and Silverman (1994). Here, we shall concentrate more on the practical tasks, rather than on theoretical issues.

Descriptive Analysis

Description and analysis of qualitative information are closely linked, hence the phrase *descriptive analysis*. This includes some *description* of the purpose of the study, the study site, and people involved which is normally presented in the introductory sections of a report. However, descriptive analysis focuses on the information gathered in relation to how it was gathered, where, and by whom. This involves reviewing the information, identifying links, patterns, and common themes, arranging the facts in order, and presenting them as they are, without adding any comments on their significance. This is usually presented in the *Results* section of a study report. The order in which the results are presented may be chronological, following the order in which the facts were obtained; or hierarchical, in order of their relative importance to the heart of the investigation. The introductory description and the descriptive analysis (results) sections of a study report should enable you to answer basic questions. For example:

Introductory Sections

- Where was the study conducted? What are the physical and climatic conditions in which people live?

- When was the study conducted? Why?

- What were the study aims, objectives, and intended outputs?

- Who conducted the study? Which methods/tools were used? Why?

- How did people participate in the study? Which ethnic, language or other groups were involved? How does the level of participation achieved in your study compare with your project's general ethos concerning (community) participation?

Results Section

What does the information gathered consist of:

- by method/tool of investigation used;

- by cluster of hygiene practices;

- by any other relevant order?

Answers to these questions require rigorous analysis and description, but not interpretation (see Box 24 for an example of how *results* are distinguished from *discussion of findings* or *interpretation*).

BOX 24

An Example to Demonstrate How Reporting Results Differs from Interpretation

In a hygiene evaluation study conducted in rural western Kenya, several methods and tools were used including mapping, Three-pile sorting, Spot-check Observations, and Semi-structured (informal) Interviews. With regard to latrine use, the findings were as follows:

Mapping
Maps created by study participants in both villages revealed that most latrines (seventeen out of twenty-one in Village 1, and twenty-five out of twenty-six in Village 2) were located outside the courtyards.

Three-Pile Sorting
The picture of a VIP latrine with a curtain which did not reach the floor (so that the feet of the person using the latrine could be seen) was categorized as *bad* in both villages.

Observations
Children's faeces were noticed in the compound only if the mother was absent. In both villages, very little faecal contamination was observed in both the domestic and the public environment.

Informal Interviews
Others reported that they normally train their young children to defecate in a specially designated place within the compound...after defecation, the child would let the mother know and she would dispose of the faeces either by taking it to the latrine (with a hoe), or by digging and burying it in the ground.

These and other findings were then put together, crosschecked and interpreted, and presented in the *Discussion* section of the report as follows:

"In the Luo culture, it is generally held that contact with human faeces is defiling and thus to be avoided at all costs...Firstly, there are clear gender-specific rules about latrine construction and maintenance...Secondly, if a latrine is to be used, and used by everyone, then it should be located appropriately...If a latrine is located within the compound, it cannot be shared by in-laws...the use of a latrine inside the compound of one's in-laws is seen by the Luo as tantamount to *undressing* or *being naked* in front of one's in-laws, even though nobody actually sees the act of undressing or the state of being naked. Such notions of nakedness relate to privacy which is a very important and well recognized requirement for latrine acceptance and use...The results of the three-pile sorting activities certainly support the privacy argument."

Sufficient detail should be included in the descriptive analysis to enable the reader to see the investigative steps you have followed, how you made methodological decisions, or changes of direction, and why. Remember that the facts have to be presented clearly, coherently, and fully before they can be interpreted. A very important feature of the descriptive analysis is the checking and crosschecking of information in order to establish the quality or trustworthiness of the findings. We shall deal with this separately in detail in "Establishing the Trustworthiness of Information."

Interpretation

The second stage is to determine what the results mean and how significant they are in the specific context to which they belong. The reasons behind certain hygiene practices and to what extent they are influenced by sociocultural factors can be teased out when the study team's multiple perspectives are brought to bear on the results. Wider issues concerning our understanding of the links between hygiene practices and health can also be explored in the light of the findings.

The following are some of the questions for the study team to answer when interpreting the study results:

■ What do the results mean?

■ Why did the results turn out the way they did?

■ What are possible explanations of the results?

■ Have all the *why* questions been answered? Do some of them require further investigation?

The interpretation of findings should ideally reflect the comments and suggestions made by members of the study population(s) during the feedback sessions that are built into the use of investigative and analytical methods/tools, such as those described in Chapters 5 and 6. This will help minimize the biases that can creep into the interpretation of results, making sure that they are not separated from the context in which information was gathered (see Box 24).

Judgement

Descriptive analysis and interpretation of results ultimately lead to judging the findings as positive or negative or both, and stating the reasons why. The values of the study team and other stakeholders are brought to bear on the study findings. For example, the findings may show what is good, bad, desirable, or undesirable in the way the project has promoted improved water supply, sanitation, and hygiene/health, in the way people have responded to external interventions, and why. The question to be answered here is:

■ What is the significance of the findings to the various stakeholders in this particular setting?

◆ to your project?

◆ to the study population?

◆ to applied researchers interested in the links between particular hygiene practices and health?

The interpretation and judgement of results are usually presented in the *Discussion* section of a report. It is important to strike a fair balance between the positive and negative aspects of the findings. For example, positive findings should be emphasized without brushing over negative ones. Similarly, negative findings should not only be listed, but discussed in a way that explores possible practical solutions or feasible remedies. The discussion section should be followed by the conclusions which may be presented in the same section or separately under *Conclusions.*

Recommendations

The fourth stage is to draw some recommendations for action to be taken on the basis of the analysis, interpretation, and judgement of study findings. The *Recommendations* section of a report normally follows the discussion and conclusions and should address the following questions.

■ What are the implications of the findings, based on your analysis, interpretation, and judgements? What are the implications:

◆ for your particular project?

◆ for other projects that may be interested to learn from your findings?

◆ for any other interested parties, such as researchers?

■ What should be done by your project and other stakeholders on the basis of the analysis, interpretation, and judgement of your study results?

The more the different concerned parties or stakeholders are involved in the interpretation and judgement of the study results, the easier it will be for you to reflect their interests in the recommendations. Practical and feasible suggestions should be clearly included in the recommendations.

Establishing the Trustworthiness of Information

As discussed in "Putting in Place Data Quality Checks" in Chapter 4, the criteria for establishing trustworthiness of qualitative data are essential components of the study design and conduct which enhance the trustworthiness (or *goodness*) of the information gathered. Unlike the statistical significance or goodness-of-fit tests applied to quantitative data, the criteria for trustworthiness of qualitative data are not a set of tests to be applied to the information after it has been collected, but in-built checks that are put in place before information gathering begins, and monitored throughout the conduct of investigation (see Chapter 4).

You should be able to judge the trustworthiness of the information you have gathered by applying all the criteria you put in place when designing the study and while conducting it. The number of criteria applied may vary from one study to another, depending on the resources (human, material, time), and other constraints on the study design and execution. However, the following key criteria constitute the minimum requirements that should be met in order to establish the trustworthiness or the quality of qualitative information.

- *Prolonged or intense engagement* of the study team with the study population. The duration of the study will be determined by resources available and the study team's familiarity with the study population. A lot can be done in a couple of weeks, especially if field workers know their study population very well. If not, a longer time will be required for the team to establish rapport with the population and minimize biases introduced by unusual manners and the unnecessary separation of the study team from the community. Be clear and honest in reporting your estimate of biases that might have crept into the study due to the type of engagement between the study team and the population(s).

- *Triangulation* of sources, methods, and investigators. As discussed in Chapter 4, it is often not feasible or practical to design a study in which means of triangulation of sources, methods, and investigators can all be put in place and applied. For example, one study may be conducted by using focus group discussions with caretakers of young children, semi-structured interviews with the same category of respondents and spot-check observations of selected households, and the study team may consist of very few individuals with similar disciplinary backgrounds. Another study may employ a larger study team with diverse backgrounds and skills and sufficient resources to enable them to use participatory investigative and analytical tools as well. Crosschecking information can be done in both cases through triangulation of sources and methods, or triangulation of methods and investigators. The most important thing is that trustworthiness of the results is checked and crosschecked by triangulation. Your report should include a clear account of the triangulation carried out.

■ *Feedback and discussion with the population.* This will help in finding possible paths for the interpretation of findings and should be documented in the report.

■ *Peer review/checking.* When peers, independent reviewers, including perhaps some of your colleagues who were not directly involved in the investigation processes, check your results, they may identify areas where you may need to provide more information or justification for the conclusions drawn. This means that your study report has to include rigorous description and analysis, with an attached *diary of activities* containing sufficient detail on when and how the study was carried out, for reference.

Peer reviews are most productive when criticisms are put to the study team clearly and constructively. However, you should be prepared to respond to difficult questions and/or not-so-constructive criticisms as well. You may need to review and, if necessary, clarify major decisions and changes of direction made during the conduct of the study. To help in preparation for such eventualities, self criticism during the processes of investigation and analysis should be encouraged among members of the study team, in an atmosphere of trust and openness.

Study reports that include very little or no detail on how the study was conducted, when, and why methodological and other decisions were made may arouse suspicion in the reviewer's mind about the trustworthiness of the findings, and may even jeopardize the investigators' credibility and status.

Presentation of Findings

The results of your hygiene evaluation study may be reported in different ways depending on the target audience or readership. To begin with, you will have a written report which will contain a complete record of the study processes and findings. Once you have completed the report, you may decide to extract parts of it, and prepare short summaries for dissemination among the various stakeholders who will expect to learn about your results. In this section, we will deal with the complete report first and then suggest additional ways in which it may be disseminated among specific audiences or readerships.

Writing a Complete Study Report

At the end of the investigation and analysis processes, you will find yourself with considerable amounts of fieldnotes, charts, and other written records of what you have done. These will all need to be systematically organized, kept in notebooks, and files compiled by hand or on a computer, if available. You can then start putting them together following a report outline, as shown in "Stages of Analysis and Interpretation of Findings" in this chapter. Box 25 provides an example of a report outline.

Writing Separate Summaries for Specific Readers or Interest Groups

You may need to send short summaries such as an executive summary to your project funders, the study population, local community groups, governmental, and/or non-governmental counterparts. It is important to balance well the positive and negative findings when reporting in short, executive summary format. By definition, an executive summary does not allow the reader the benefit of seeing the findings in the context. Evaluation study results are seldom entirely positive or entirely negative, but a combination of the two. Whether they are interpreted as positive or negative depends on who is interpreting and using them.

You may also want to prepare short articles summarizing your findings for dissemination in local and/or regional networks of practitioners working in the fields of health/hygiene education, water supply, and sanitation; research networks such as the global applied research network (GARNET) which has a topic network on Hygiene Behaviour, the working group on Promotion of Sanitation, and so on. You will need to bear in mind the interests of each of these groups when deciding what to include, and what language and style to use.

Making Verbal Presentations to Selected Groups and Inviting Their Comments and Suggestions

You may find it beneficial to present partial or full results of your investigation to some of the most important stakeholders in the study in order to elicit their responses to the analysis and interpretation of your findings. For example, in Chapters 5 and 6, we looked at a number of participatory tools for information gathering (mapping, historyline, seasonal calendars, pocket chart) which included the presentation of information gathered to the study participants there and then. Charts, graphs, and other visual displays can be used to present the findings in ways that will interest and stimulate participants. However, only overall results should be given and not details of individual interviews or households.

BOX 25
Outline of a Report

- Title page: Authors' Names, Institutions, and Date
- Executive Summary (this is written last—after the report has been completed)
- Acknowledgments
- Table of Contents
- Lists of Tables and Figures
- List of People consulted/List of Abbreviations/Glossary (as appropriate)
- Introduction (including background to study and organization of the report)
- Study Design and Organization
  - Study aims, objectives, and intended outputs
  - Description of study team
  - Study schedule
  - Training
- Study Site(s) and Population(s)
  - Background (including maps of study sites)
  - Sampling strategies
- Methods and Tools Used for Investigation and Analysis
- Results (including descriptive analysis but no interpretation)
- Discussion (including interpretation and judgement of findings)
- Appraisal of Methods/Tools Used
- Conclusions and Recommendations
- References (a list of any documentary materials used and referred to in the report)
- Appendices/Annexes (these may include details of the study schedule; complete diary of activities; observation and interview schedules used; fieldnotes such as transcriptions of interviews, and anything else judged to be relevant to the contents of the report but is too bulky to be included in the main body of the report.)

Your project may already have trained personnel (e.g., trainer or project spokesperson) who can present the study findings at workshops, meetings and conferences where various audiences may be interested in hearing about your findings.

The type of visual and other materials you can use to present your results will depend on the resources available. Often, summaries of findings written on flip-charts using thick marker pens and big letters (including diagrams, charts, and graphs where appropriate) are the most effective ways to present findings to large groups in both rural and urban areas. These require less financial resources to prepare and can be more creative and fun to do.

Organizing a Discussion or Debate on the Findings in Which Opposing Points of View Can Be Aired

This is a particularly good idea if the level of participation of the different stakeholders is high and if your findings are likely to be interpreted significantly different by groups according to their opposing interests. In the final analysis, comparisons must be made carefully and appropriately to avoid the drawing of wrong conclusions.

Implementation of Findings

Many of the methods and tools described in this handbook lead naturally from collecting and analysing data (i.e., establishing what the problem is) to planning what needs to be done to address the issues raised. For example, a healthwalk may reveal that part of a community is using a water source particularly vulnerable to pollution for its drinking water. Indeed, we have seen in Chapter 5 the impact of information gathered during a healthwalk on project design and implementation. Similarly, information from focus group discussions and semi-structured interviews may reveal a higher incidence of diarrhoea among this group. Presentation of these findings to the community will almost inevitably lead to a discussion of what needs to be done to remedy the situation, moving the emphasis from data collection to implementation. Thus a hygiene evaluation study does not end with the presentation of findings. It should lead to follow-up action on the basis of the findings.

Whether or not participatory approaches are given importance in the evaluation, the end result of the study will be the identification of *high risk* hygiene practices which currently exist, embedded in a context of local physical conditions, beliefs, and ideas. You will almost inevitably advocate that follow up action should include hygiene promotion activities. The goal of any hygiene promotion project must be to influence people to abandon the high risk practices identified in favour of low risk, safe practices. But, what influences people's decisions to change their normal practice? Many studies have shown that the answer to this question is "not received knowledge alone." Commonly, four factors influencing behavioural change are identified:

- *Facilitation.* The new practice makes life easier for the person adopting it.

- *Understanding.* The new practice makes sense in the context of existing local knowledge/ideas.

- *Approval.* Important and respected people in the community approve of and have adopted the practice.

- *Ability to make change.* It is physically possible for the person concerned to make the necessary changes.

Below are some examples of how information gathered using this handbook may be fed into an implementation process that takes these four factors into account:

Facilitation. In order to get people to use safe water for drinking purposes, it may be necessary to ensure that there are sufficient protected water sources throughout the community to make it easier and more convenient to use as opposed to traditional, unprotected ones. In planning terms, this may mean continuing a mapping exercise that identified existing sources instead of using the map, with the community, to plan the location of new water points.

Understanding. Hygiene promotion messages and activities are not received by people in a vacuum. Rather they are assessed, accepted, modified, or rejected by people within the context of their existing health concerns and beliefs about illness. A number of similar evaluations have, for example, elicited the local concepts of *hot* and *cold* illnesses that need to be treated by controlling diet and reducing intake of some foods. In a number of cases, the promotion of ORS has run into difficulties because diarrhoea is classified as a *hot* illness requiring treatment with cooling substances, while sugar, a major constituent of ORS, is categorized as *hot*, therefore rendering ORS an unsuitable treatment. Project implementers have found various ways to overcome such problems including substituting honey (considered a cooling substance) for sugar in one case, and in another, encouraging people to use ORS in conjunction with herbal teas made from guava leaves—a traditional remedy considered *cooling* and seen to overcome the perceived *heating* effect of the sugar in ORS.

Approval. In order to enhance the desirability of change, it may be necessary to target hygiene promotion at certain groups of trend setters, such as traditional healers, local leaders, or young mothers who are likely to be copied by their peers. Often this would best be done through a continued use of the group discussion techniques used earlier in the evaluation.

Ability. If behavioural change requires resources, it may be beyond some people's abilities to make the change. Promotion of latrines, for example, may need careful planning with communities, using many of the techniques discussed earlier to enable targeted assistance/subsidies to be allocated to those who would otherwise be unable to make the change.

In projects where the promotion of *low risk* hygiene practices has been achieved, the follow-up action to evaluations may involve tackling other issues that are next in the list of priorities. Whatever the outcomes of your study are, we shall be interested to learn about your experiences of using this handbook (see Evaluation Sheet at the back of the book).

Selected Reading

Planning

Feuerstein MT. 1986. *Partners in Evaluation.* Macmillan, London. Distributors: Macmillan and TALC (Teaching Aids at Low Cost), PO Box 49, St. Albans, Hertfordshire AL1 4AX, UK.

Folmer HR, Moynihan MN and Schothorst PM. 1992. *Testing and Evaluating Manuals.* International Health Learning Materials (HLM) Programme, World Health Organization, Geneva. Distributor: WHO (HLM), 1211, Geneva 27, Switzerland.

Moser CON. 1993. *Gender Planning and Development: Theory, practice and training.* Routledge, London. Distributors: Routledge, 11 New Fetter Lane, London EC4P 4EE, UK.

Murray Bradley S. 1995. *How People Use Pictures.* International Institute for Environment and Development, London. Distributor: IIED, London.

Overseas Development Administration 1995. *Guidance note on how to do stakeholder analysis of aid projects and programmes.* Overseas Development Administration (ODA), Social Development Department, London. Distributor: ODA, 94 Victoria Street, London, SW1E 5JL, UK.

Srinivasan L. 1992. *Options for Educators: A Monograph for Decision Makers on Alternative Participatory Strategies.* PACT/CDS, Communications Development Service, New York. Distributor: PACT, Inc, 777 UN Plaza, New York, New York 10017, USA.

White A. 1981. "Community Participation in Water and Sanitation." Technical Paper Series No. 17, IRC International Water and Sanitation Centre, The Hague, The Netherlands.

Methods

Bentley ME, Boot MT, Gittelsohn J, Stallings R. 1994. "The use of structured observations in the study of health behaviour." IRC Occasional Paper No. 27, London School of Hygiene & Tropical Medicine and IRC, The Hague. Distributor: IRC, PO Box 93190, 2509 AD The Hague, The Netherlands. This can be obtained free of charge and if necessary photocopied as specified in its copyright statement.

Boot M, Cairncross S, eds. 1993. *Actions Speak: The study of hygiene behaviour in water and sanitation projects.* LSHTM and IRC, The Hague. Distributor: IRC, PO Box 93190, 2509 AD The Hague, The Netherlands. This is not free, but concessions may be agreed where applicable.

Cairncross S, Kochar V, eds. 1994. *Studying Hygiene Behaviour: Methods, issues and experience.* Sage, New Delhi. Distributor: Sage Publications, 32 M-Block Market, Greater Kailash-I, New Delhi 110048, India/6, Bonhill Street, London EC2A, 4PU, UK/ 2455 Teller Road, Thousand Oaks, California 91320, USA.

Dawson S, Manderson L, Tallo V. 1993. *The Focus Groups Manual.* INFDC, Boston. Distributors: International Nutrition Foundation for Developing Countries (INFDC), PO Box 500, Charles Street Station, Boston, MA 01224-0500, USA.

Herman E, Bentley M. 1993. *Rapid Assessment Procedures (RAP): To improve the household management of diarrhea.* Methods for Social Research in Disease, International Nutrition Foundation for Developing Countries, Boston. Distributor: INFDC (as above).

Kolb DA. 1984. *Experiential Learning: Experience as a source of learning and development.* Prentice-Hall, New Jersey.

Narayan D. 1993. "Participatory Evaluation: Tools for managing change in water and sanitation." World Bank Technical Paper, Number 207, Washington, DC. Distributor: The World Bank, 1818 H Street, NW, Washington, DC 20433, USA.

Participatory Rural Appraisal Handbook: Conducting PRAs in Kenya. Natural Resources Management Support Series, No. 1, National Environment Secretariat, Nairobi.

Patton MQ. 1990. *Qualitative Evaluation and Research Methods.* (second edition) Sage, London.

Pelto PJ, Pelto GH. 1978. *Anthropological Research: The structure of inquiry.* Cambridge University Press, New York. Distributor: Cambridge University Press, 40 West 20th Street, New York, NY 10011, USA.

Scrimshaw NS, Gleason GR, eds. 1992. *Rapid Assessment Procedures: Qualitative Methodologies for Planning and Evaluation of Health Related Programmes.* INFDC, Boston. Distributor: INFDC (as above).

Scrimshaw S, Hurtado E. 1987. *Rapid Assessment Procedures for Nutrition and Primary Health Care.* UCLA Latin American Centre, Los Angeles.

Srinivasan L. 1990. *Tools for Community Participation: A Manual for training trainers in participatory techniques.* PROWWESS/UNDP Technical Series, Involving Women in Water and Sanitation, United Nations Development Programme, New York. Distributor: (as above).

Analysis and Interpretation of Data

Gill GJ. 1993. *O.K., The data's lousy, but it's all we've got.* Gatekeeper Series No. 38, International Institute for Environment and Development, London.

Miles MB, Huberman AM. 1994. *Qualitative Data Analysis.* Sage, London.

Patton MQ. 1986. *Utilization-focused Evaluation.* Sage, London.

Pretty JN. 1994. "Alternative systems of inquiry for a sustainable agriculture." *Inst Dev Studies Bull* 25:37–48.

Silvermann D. 1994. *Interpreting Qualitative Data.* Sage, London. Distributor: Sage (as above).

Water Supply and Sanitation

Bern C, Martines J, de Zoysa I, Glass R. 1992. "The magnitude of the global problem of diarrhoeal disease: a ten-year update." *Bull WHO* 70:707–714.

Cairncross S, Feachem R. 1993. *Environmental Health Engineering in the Tropics.* 2d ed. John Wiley & Sons, Chichester. Distributors: Macmillan and TALC (as above).

Morgan P. 1990. *Rural Water Supplies and Sanitation.* Blair Research Laboratory & Ministry of Health, Harare. Distributor: MacMillan (as above).

Simpson-Herbert M. 1983. *Methods for Gathering Sociocultural Data for Water Supply and Sanitation Projects.* UNDP/World Bank, Technology Advisory Group (TAG), Washington, D.C.

Wagner EG, Lanoix JN. 1958. *Excreta Disposal for Rural Areas and Small Communities.* WHO, Monograph Series, No. 39, World Health Organization, Geneva.

Warren KS, Bundy D, Anderson R, Davis AR, Henderson DA, Jamison DT, Prescott N, Senft A. 1991. Helminth infection. In: Jamison DT, Mosley WH, eds. *Evolving health-sector priorities in developing countries.* World Bank, Washington, DC.

WASH Project. 1993. *Lessons learned in water, sanitation and health: thirteen years of experience in developing countries.* Water and Sanitation for Health Project, Arlington, VA.

World Health Organization. 1983. *Minimum Evaluation Procedure (MEP) for water supply and sanitation projects.* WHO, Geneva. Distributor: WHO, Rural Environmental Health, Geneva.

Hygiene Promotion

Boot M. 1991. *Just Stir Gently: The way to mix hygiene education with water supply and sanitation.* IRC, The Hague. Distributor: IRC (as above).

Hubley J. 1993. *Communicating Health: An action guide to health education and health promotion.* Macmillan, London. Distributors: Macmillan and TALC (as above).

World Health Organization. 1993a. "Improving water and sanitation hygiene behaviours for the reduction of diarrhoeal disease." Report of an informal consultation, WHO/CWS & CDD, Geneva. Distributor: WHO, Rural Environmental Health.

World Health Organization. 1993b. "New directions for hygiene and sanitation promotion: The findings of a regional informal consultation." WHO, Regional Office for South-East Asia, New Delhi and CWS, Geneva.

Yacoob M, Braddy B, Edwards L. 1992. "Rethinking Sanitation, Adding behavioural change to the project mix." WASH Technical Report No. 72, Arlington. Distributor: Environmental Health Project, 1611 N. Kent St., Room 1001, Arlington, VA 22209-2111, USA.

EVALUATION SHEET

(Please use additional paper if your answers require more space than is provided)

About Yourself

1. Name:

   Position held and project's name:

   Address:

2. Who introduced you to this handbook and what made you decide to read/use it?

About This Handbook

1. Was the language clear and easy to understand?

2. Which section(s) of the handbook did you find easiest to understand and which parts were most difficult?

3. What do you think should have been included to make this handbook more useful to you?

4. Which sections did you think could have been left out?

5. Do you think this handbook should be translated into another language(s)? If so, which one(s)?

About Your Hygiene Evaluation Study

1. Describe each member of your study team including position/title, gender, and language(s) used during the investigation.

2. Which questions did your hygiene evaluation aim to investigate?

3. What was/were your working hypothesis/es?

4. Which methods and tools did you use?

5. What difficulties did you encounter?

6. Which level of participation was achieved?

7. What were your main findings?

8. Which of these findings were unexpected/surprising?

9. Who will use these findings? When?

10. How much of the information you obtained do you think could have gathered without using this handbook?

Tear off this sheet along the perforations and send it (along with any additional papers) to the following address:

Astier Almedom, LSHTM, Keppel St., London WC1E 7HT, U.K. Fax: +44 171 636 7843